F

and Dermatology

The Foot: Problems in Podiatry and Dermatology

Rodney Dawber
Consultant Dermatologist
The Churchill Hospital
Oxford, UK

Ivan Bristow
Podiatrist, Dermatology Department
The Churchill Hospital
Oxford, UK

Jean Mooney
Senior Teacher
The London Foot Hospital
London, UK

MARTIN DUNITZ

The views expressed are those of the authors and are not necessarily those of Sandoz Pharmaceutical Division.

First published in the United Kingdom
in 1996 by
Martin Dunitz Ltd
The Livery House
7–9 Pratt Street
London NW1 0AE

A CIP record for this book is available from the British Library.

ISBN 1-85317-405-X

Printed and bound in Spain by Cayfosa

Contents

Anatomy of the foot and nail

Introduction

The human foot is a complex structure, made up of 28 bones, including two sesamoid bones, and 40 joints, with 12 extrinsic and 19 intrinsic muscles. The foot has two main functions: to act as a flexible support to the lower limb; and to act as a rigid lever to help propulsion during locomotion.

Faults in the interrelationship of these structures can cause changes to the surface soft tissues, including nail disorders; such faults may also alter the symptoms and signs of other diseases affecting the foot and nails.

The bones and principal joints of the foot are shown in Figure 1; the most important joints in the foot are: the ankle; the subtalar joint (STJ); the midtarsal joint (MTJ) and the first metatarsophalangeal joint (1 MTPJ).

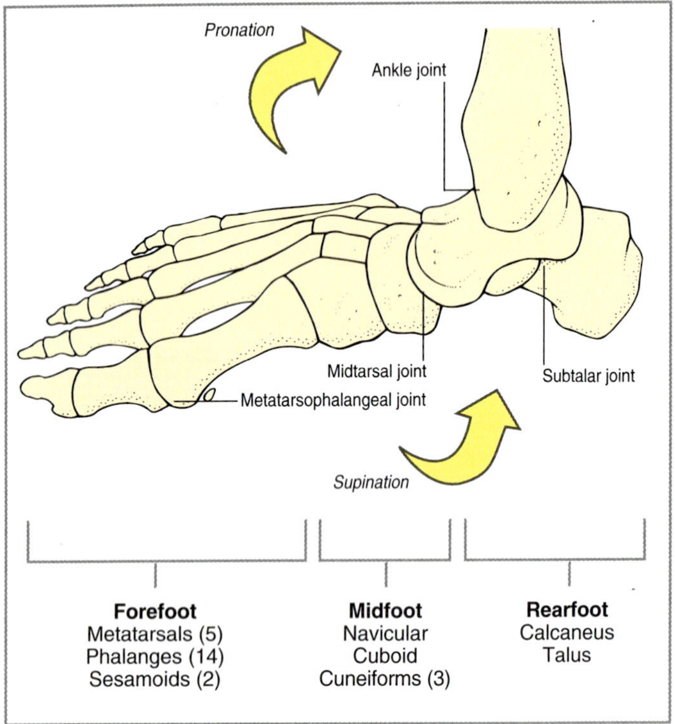

Figure 1
The bone and principal joints of the foot.

The foot supinates just before the heel makes contact with the ground, becomes pronated in the middle of the footstep, and supinates again at toe-off (Figure 2). The pronated foot is flexible and will adapt to the ground surface, whereas the supinated foot is rigid and acts as a lever aiding efficient locomotion (see also gait cycle diagram, Figure 10, page 18).

Problems can occur in the foot associated with excessive joint movement; these are shown in Table 1.

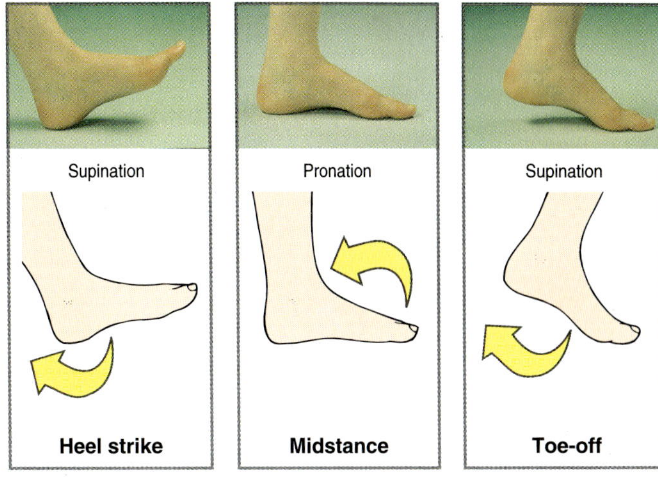

Figure 2
The positions of the foot during walking.

Excess pronation movement	Foot problems arising	Associated problems
Excess pronation at the STJ and MTJ	Flat foot	Tarsal coalition
	Chronic foot strain	
	Hallux rigidus	Dorsal bunion
Lateral movement of the hallux	Hallux abductovalgus	Nail problems Medial bunion Metatarsalgia
	Lesser toe deformities	Corns and callouses Interdigital maceration Interdigital fungal infections

Table 1
Foot problems associated with excessive joint movement

Muscles controlling foot movement

Foot movements are controlled by the extrinsic muscles in the lower leg and intrinsic muscles within the foot (see Tables 2 and 3, and Figure 3).

Group	Action on foot	Muscles
Posterior group	Plantar-flexion at ankle	Gastrocnemius, soleus, plantaris, tibialis posterior, flexor hallucis longus, flexor digitorum longus
Anterior group	Dorsiflexion of the ankle	Tibialis anterior, extensor hallucis longus, extensor digitorum longus, peroneus tertius
Lateral group	Eversion of the foot	Peroneus longus, peroneus brevis
Pronators	Pronation of the foot and plantar-flexion of the first metatarsal	Peroneus longus, peroneus brevis
Supinators	Supination of the foot and inversion of the foot	Tibialis posterior, tibialis anterior

Table 2
The muscles of the lower limb which control foot movement (the extrinsic muscles)

Site	Layer	Muscle	Action
Dorsal	—	Extensor digitorum brevis	Dorsiflex and abduct toes at MTPJs
Plantar	1	Flexor digitorum brevis	Plantar-flex toes 2, 3, 4, 5 and MTPJs Reinforces long arch of foot
		Abductor hallucis	Plantar-flexes and abducts hallux (away from midline of body)
	2	Abductor digit minimi	Abducts little toe (towards midline of body)
		Flexor accessorius/ Quadratus plantae	Plantar-flexes lesser toes Augments pull of flexor digitorum longus
		Lubricales	Plantar-flex 2, 3, 4, 5 MTPJs Dorsiflex IPJs toes 2,3,4,5
		Flexor hallucis brevis	Plantar-flexes 1 MTPJ and abducts hallux (away from midline of body)
		Adductor hallucis (oblique)	Plantar-flexes 1 MPTJ and abducts hallux (away from midline of body)
		Adductor hallucis (transverse)	Accentuates transverse arch at MTPJs
	3	Flexor digiti minimi brevis	Plantar-flexes 5 MTPJ
	4	Plantar interossei	Abduct toes 3, 4, 5 (away from midline of body)
		Dorsal interossei	Adduct toes 2, 3, 4 (towards midline of foot) Plantar-flex 2, 3, 4 MTPJs

IPJ, interphalangeal joint; 2, 3, 4, 5 MTPJ, fifth metatarsophalangeal joint.

Table 3
The intrinsic muscles of the foot which control foot movement

If the foot is malaligned, the intrinsic muscles (Figure 4) may not be strong enough to overcome the joint distortion imposed by the extrinsic muscles.

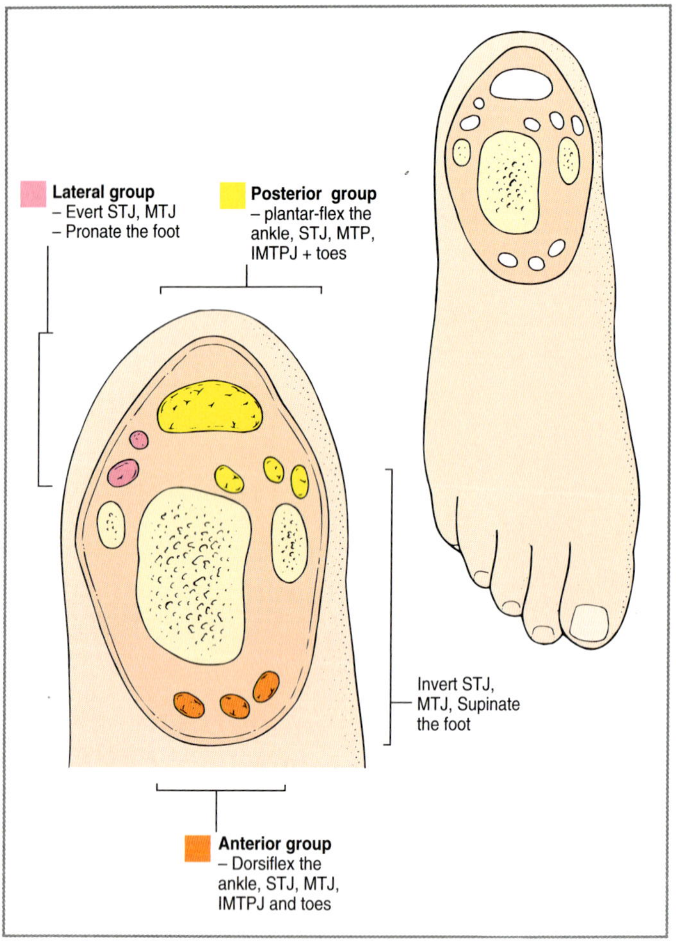

Figure 3

Cross-section of the lower limb at the ankle to show the extrinsic muscles of the foot.

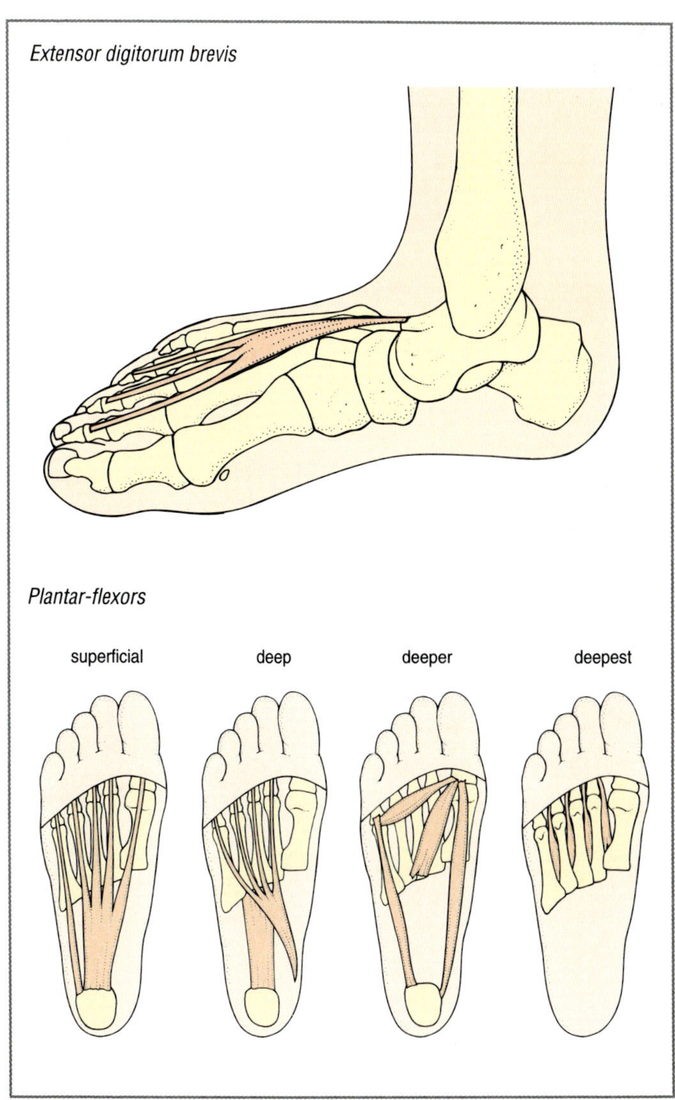

Figure 4
Intrinsic foot muscles.

Vasculature of the foot

The arterial system

The arterial supply of the foot and an individual toe are shown in Figure 5, with an indication of the pulses found in the foot.

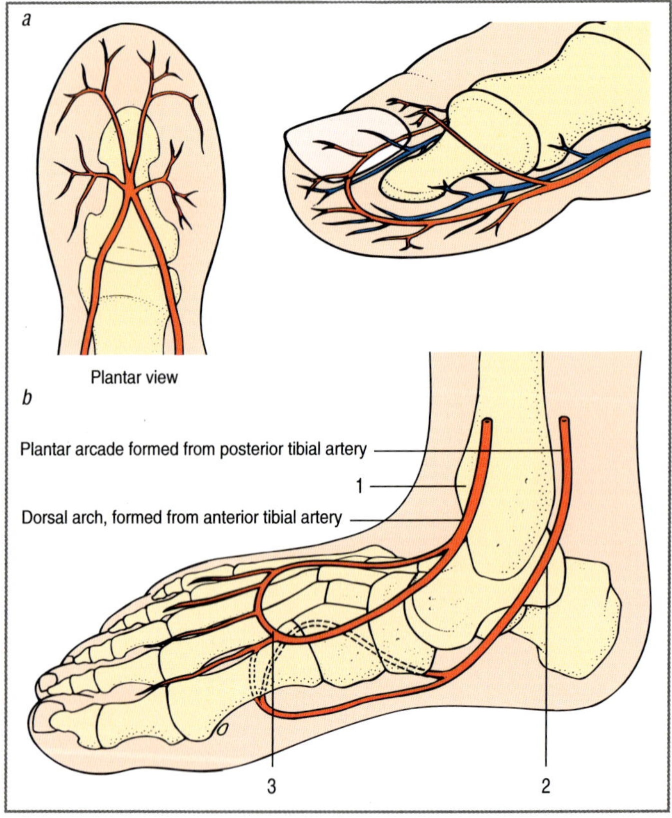

Figure 5

The arterial supply of (a) the toe and (b) the foot. Arteries in the foot:

1. Anterior tibial

2. Posterior tibial (tibialis posterior)

3. Dorsal (dorsalis pedis)

The venous system

The venous drainage of the foot is by three principal veins as shown in Table 4.

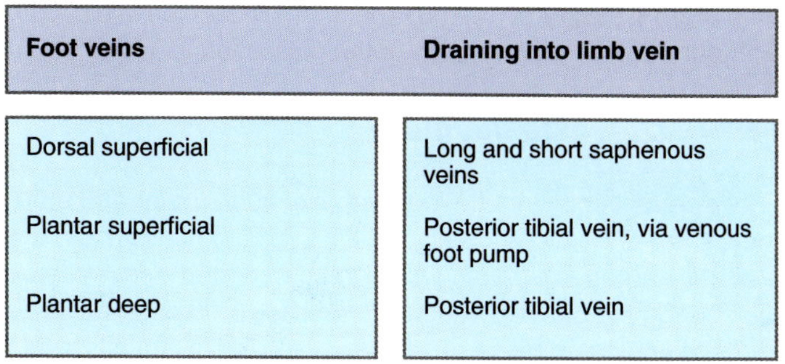

Foot veins	Draining into limb vein
Dorsal superficial	Long and short saphenous veins
Plantar superficial	Posterior tibial vein, via venous foot pump
Plantar deep	Posterior tibial vein

Table 4
Venous drainage of the foot

The venous foot pump (Figure 6) is active during walking; at toe-off, the deep veins are compressed and emptied by contraction of the extrinsic and intrinsic plantar muscles, thus propelling blood proximally and up the lower leg.

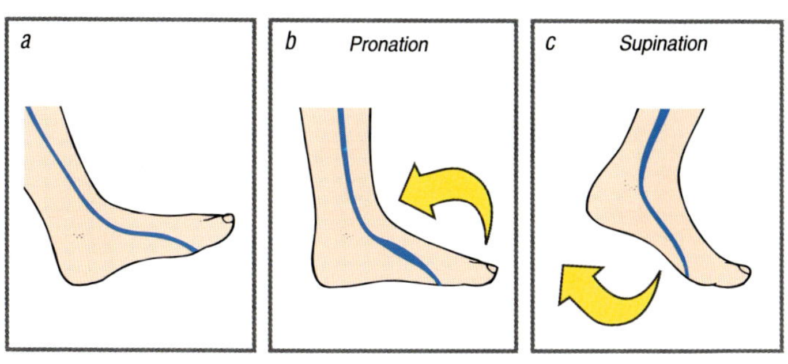

Figure 6
The venous foot pump: (a) plantar veins drain into the great saphenous vein; (b) plantar veins extend with pronation of foot; and (c) plantar veins empty with supination of foot.

Lymphatic drainage of the foot

The lymphatic drainage occurs on the lateral side of the foot into the popliteal nodes, and on the medial side of the foot into the inguinal nodes.

Nerve supply to the foot

The nerves supplying the foot carry sensory, motor and autonomic fibres. The dermoepidermal junction of the skin and the nail bed areas are particularly well innervated with sensory fibres, and the nail bed contains many neurovascular bodies – glomus bodies; in these units some vascular dilatation occurs in response to cold, thus helping to maintain distal vascular perfusion. The distribution of dorsal and plantar dermatomes is shown in Figure 7.

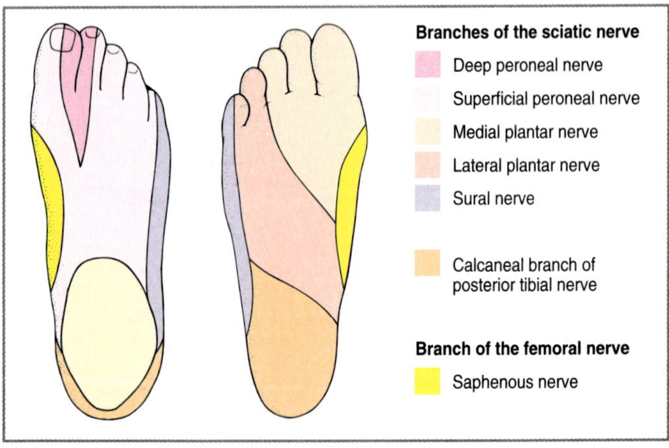

Figure 7
Dorsal and plantar dermatomes.

Fascial structures

The fasciae of the foot are divided into dorsal and plantar areas and have the characteristics shown in Table 5.

Joints are held in alignment by fibrous capsules strengthened by collateral ligaments. Both sudden injury and chronic overstretching, such as overpronation, can cause strain or sprain of ligaments. A severe sprain can cause avulsion of the ligament away from the bone.

Site	Type	Characteristics
Dorsal fascia	Superficial	Thin, little subcuticular fat Forms retinacula at dorsum of ankle Forms medial and lateral collateral ligaments of ankle Subject to adventitious bursa formation
Plantar fascia	Superficial	Thick, especially under heel and MTPJs Fibrofatty meshwork Acts as a shock absorber Lost or reduced in elderly people and in ischaemia Drifts up under toes with forefoot deformities Subject to adventitious bursa formation
	Deep	Tough, fibrous, inelastic Maintains longitudinal and transverse arches Forms longitudinal and transverse ligaments of sole Subject to chronic strain in flat foot, and overpronation

Table 5
Fasciae of the foot

Skin structure

The dermis overlays the superficial fascia; it is rich in nerves and vascular plexus. Skin appendages (sweat glands, pilosebaceous units and apocrine glands) invaginate deep into the dermis.

The dorsal epidermis (Figure 8) is thin and flexible, whereas that of the plantar surface is tough and covered with a thick keratinous layer, especially in weight-bearing areas.

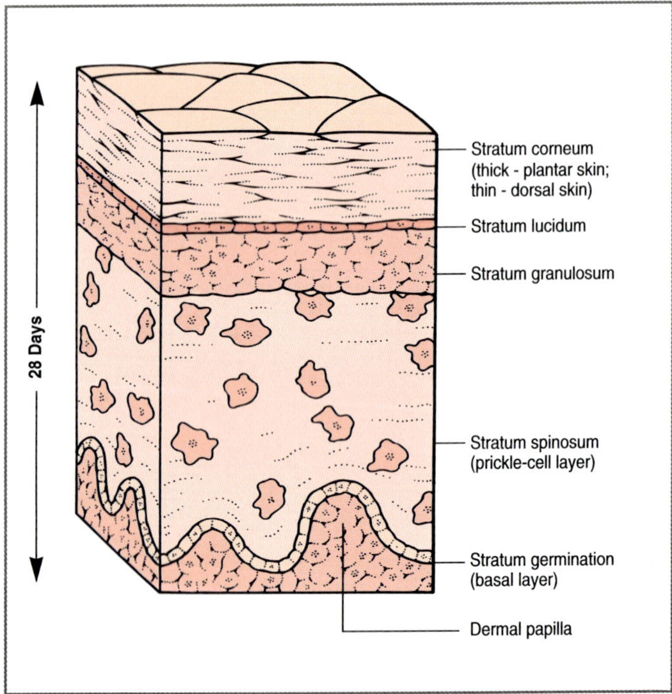

Figure 8
Structure of the epidermis.

It takes about 28 days for basal epidermal cells to move up and away (differentiate) from the germinal layer, to be shed as squames from the outer surface of the epidermis. In corn and callous formation, there is both a local increase in cell production and a decrease in the normal rate of desquamation. In normal circumstances, skin will heal readily following trauma because its normal function is to be constantly regenerated throughout life. In conditions of ulceration, this facility is considerably impaired.

The skin of the foot will be affected by force of any type, and some of the effects are given in Table 6.

Force	Type	Effects on skin
Sudden, severe	Friction, shear	Loss/tearing of epidermis/dermis Exposure of subcuticular and underlying tissues
Moderate, repeated	Friction, shear	Blister–acantholysis–especially in sweaty skin Callous formation
	Compression	Corn formation Ulceration and tissue breakdown
	Tension	Fissuring Seed corn formation (especially in dry skin)
Low-grade intermittent (also atopic reaction, inflammation, psoriasis)	Any of the above	Hyperkeratosis – increased cell production/decreased desquamation Parakeratosis – imperfect keratin formation/increased rate of epidermal cell turnover

Table 6
Effects of forces at skin surface

Specialized structures of the skin

Nails develop at the termini of the dorsal aspects of all digits; together with hair follicles they form the main epidermal appendages of the dorsal skin of the foot. The structure of the nail unit is indicated in Table 7 and Figure 9. Sweat glands are found in great numbers in both dorsal and plantar skin.

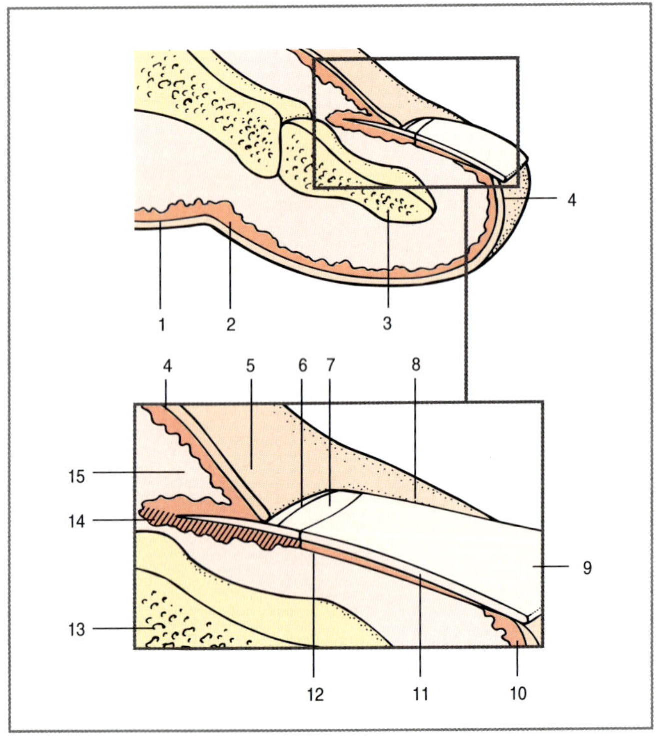

Figure 9
The nail unit.

1 Epidermis
2 Dermis
3 Bone – terminal phalanx
4 Epidermis
5 Posterior or proximal nail fold
6 Cuticle
7 Lunula
8 Lateral nail fold
9 Free margin
10 Hyponychium
11 Nail plate
12 Nail bed
13 Bone – terminal phalanx
14 Matrix (shaded area)
15 Proximal nail fold

Part	Details
Nail plate	Normally thin and translucent keratin plate; becomes discoloured, thickened and fragile with fungal infections Close adherence to nail bed and to phalangeal bone; adherence lost by trauma, and in some disease states
Proximal nail fold	Contains proximal part of nail plate Shape of fold dictates shape of forming plate Shape altered by scarring, trauma, inflammation, disease
Cuticle	Extension of dorsal epidermal stratum corneum on to nail plate seals proximal nail fold, preventing 'access' to nail matrix of organisms, irritants and potential allergens Loss of seal may lead to chronic infection (paronychia) and plate dystrophy
Matrix	Lines proximal nail fold and forms lunula Generates nail plate tissue Dermatological diseases affect matrix, causing loss of generation of normal nail plate
Lateral folds	Soft tissue sulci either side of nail plate Subject to corn/callous formation (onychophosis) and trauma (ingrowing toenail), especially with overpronation of STJ and in hypermobile foot.

Table 7
The nail unit

Unusual anatomy of nail can indicate the presence of systemic disease. The presence of hair can indicate the quality of the arterial supply to the skin (loss of hair with impaired arterial perfusion), but the amount of hair is genetically influenced. Sweat production occurs at a low level at all times, but can be increased or decreased by the factors shown in Table 8.

Activity	Condition	Exacerbated by	Skin problem
Overactivity	Hyperhidrosis	High environmental temperature	Maceration Blisters Fissures Fungal infections
	Bromhidrosis	Bacterial activity	As above
	Keratolysis	Bacterial activity	Sore sweaty erosions on soles
Underactivity	Anhidrosis	Autonomic neuropathy Ischaemia	Dry skin Tissue breakdown Seed corns

Table 8
Sweat gland activity

Foot function

Normal

The gait cycle (Figure 10) is a sequence of events of which foot function forms one part. The aim of human locomotion is to be an energy-efficient process that allows smooth movement. The function of a foot is governed by its anatomical structures and their interrelationship during movement. During the gait cycle the foot is able to exhibit two opposing features: a stable platform for propulsion and support at heel strike, and flexibility to disperse the forces generated by locomotion while simultaneously adapting to the terrain under foot.

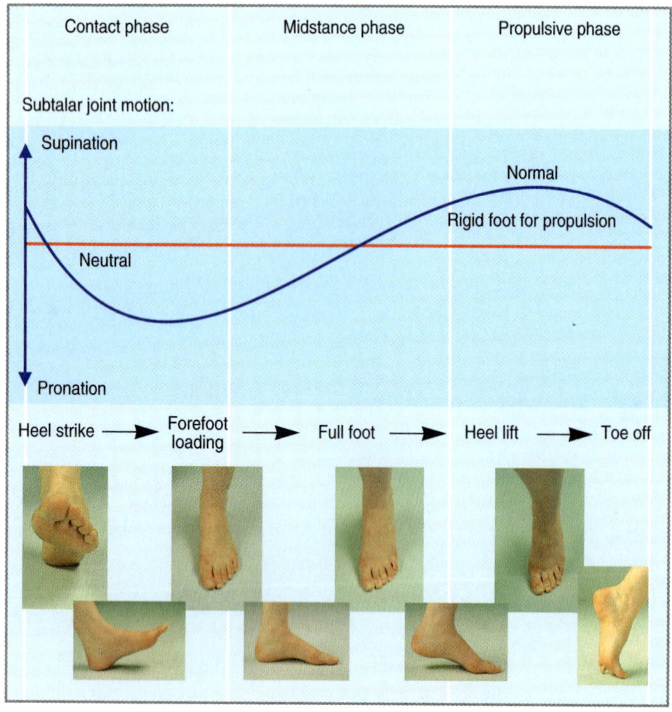

Figure 10
The position of the foot during normal gait cycle.

The change in flexibility of the foot is brought about primarily by the position of the subtalar joint (STJ) and the midtarsal joint (MTJ). At heel strike, the STJ pronates to achieve flexibility and shock absorption as the foot reaches the ground. Subtalar pronation is a movement in three body planes consisting of

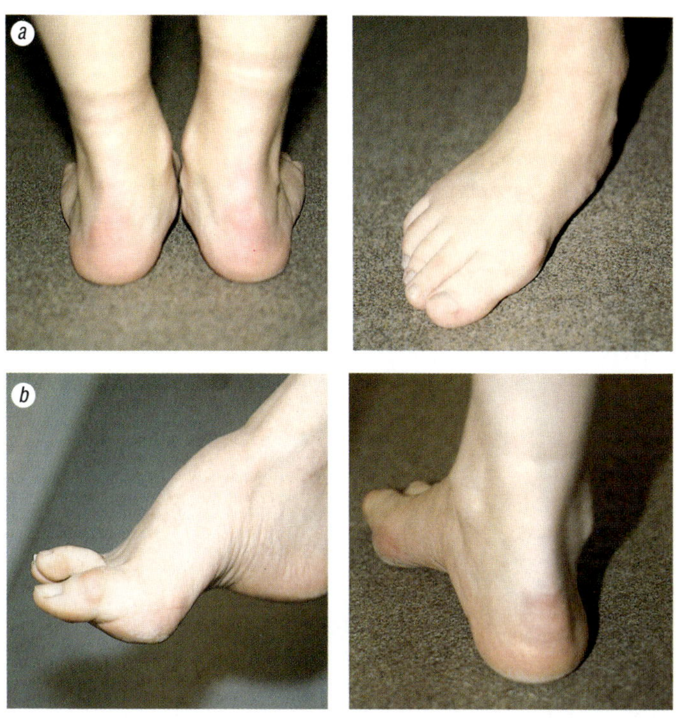

Figure 11
Features which may accompany a pronated (a) and supinated (b) foot. (a) Pronated (flat foot/pes planus): calcaneum everted, low arch, flexible or rigid foot, adductovarus toes, medial bulging of talar head, callus under 2nd, 3rd and 4th metatarsal heads. (b) Supinated (high arched foot/pes cavus): calcaneum inverted, high arch, rigid foot, clawed or retracted toes, prominent extensor tendons, callus under 1st and 5th metatarsal heads.

eversion, dorsiflexion and abduction. The effect of this pronation is to unlock the midtarsal joint and render the foot as a flexible cushion (Figure 11). Clinically, it is seen as a flat foot, with eversion of the calcaneum and lowering of the longitudinal arch of the foot slightly increasing its length.

As the foot comes into full ground contact (midstance phase), supporting the body as the opposite limb swings through, it becomes less pronated and moves into a supinated position. Supination is the reverse movement to pronation, giving the foot a more arched appearance (a triplanar movement of inversion, plantar-flexion and adduction). Subtalar joint supination allows the foot to become more rigid for effective propulsion. As the heel lifts, the foot remains in a supinated position and body weight is shifted on to the toes as the foot propulses into swing phase. A supinated,or cavus, foot is recognized by an increase in arch height, calcaneal inversion and a shortening in foot length.

Toe function is important for normal gait, especially that of the big toe, allowing smooth transmission of weight from one foot to another. As the heel lifts from the ground the intrinsic muscles stabilize the toes on the metatarsal heads to prevent buckling of the toes as the long flexor and extensor tendons function around them.

Abnormal

Abnormal foot function may arise as a result of excessive / prolonged pronation or supination occurring during the gait cycle. Pathological / excessive pronation and supination can arise as a result of malalignment in the lowerlimb, pelvis and back. Furthermore, excessive pronation or supination can trigger other problems in the foot and leg. In such cases it is pertinent to undertake biomechanical evaluation of the patient in order to elicit the cause of the problem. Table 9 summarizes some of the more common causes of abnormal pronation and supination.

Causes	Examples
Biomechanical malalignments	Forefoot inversions/eversions Tibial varum, femoral torsions Ankle equinus Pes cavus Flat foot
Congenital deformity/ inherited foot shape	Vertical talus, talipes Tarsal coalition
Neurological deficits	Cerebrovascular accidents, Charcot–Marie–Tooth disease Poliomyelitis, spina bifida Diabetic neuroarthropathy
Connective tissue disorders/ligamentous laxity	Rheumatoid arthritis Systemic lupus erythematousus

Table 9
Common causes of abnormal supination and pronation

Detrimental effects of footwear

A foot that functions abnormally, coupled with an unsuitable style of footwear can often provoke even further foot problems. These are often observed in the forefoot around the toes and particularly the toenails. Poor footwear is a major contributor to traumatic toenail pathologies and should always be assessed as well as the presenting pathology. The wearing of badly fitting footwear over a period of time can have a major moulding effect on the forefoot and should never be underestimated.

A functionally suitable shoe should exhibit the following:

- Low heel
- Suitable fastening
- A wide and deep toe box design
- Seamless interior

Assessment of the shoes should include inspection of the inside of the shoe. Tears or rub spots can often be felt in the lining, giving clues to foot function, and enlightening the clinician to its likely effects.

High-heeled footwear (usually without a suitable fastening) allows the foot to slip forward into the toe box area of the shoe, compressing and traumatizing the toes and the toenails. Long-term wearing of high heels can also lead to shortening of the Achilles tendon, characterized by pain in the calf when the patient returns to flat-heeled shoes.

With a reduction in heel height and the incorporation of lacing, or a Velcro strap, the amount of forward movement in the shoe will be reduced, holding the foot firmly back into the heel of the shoe. A toe box which is too narrow or too shallow will place undue pressure on the forefoot, this force being magnified many times during normal walking. When a patient wears these shoes, any bulging of the toe box caused by prominent toes is likely to pinpoint the source of a problem.

Shoes that are too long or without a fastening can often lead to increased nail trauma. As the foot moves around excessively in the shoe, the wearer will subconsciously claw the toes to maintain an element of stability. In doing so pressure is then borne on the dorsum and apex of the digit and nail plate.

Orthopaedic foot and nail disorders

Corns and callosities

These appear as yellowish thickened patches of epidermis most commonly seen on the feet in response to intermittent pressure or friction. They appear most frequently under the metatarsal heads, on the apices and dorsum of toes, on the lateral borders of the feet. The amount of pain experienced can range from minimal to disabling. A corn is considered to be an advanced callus having a central nucleus of hyperkeratotic skin. Corns may often be misdiagnosed as plantar warts (Table 10).

Débridement and enucleation of painful hyperkeratotic lesions gives much relief. Caustic or keratolytic medications applied to the lesions have limited value unless the cause of the underlying pressure is addressed. Most commonly hyperkeratosis results from abnormal foot function or unsuitable footwear, so redressing these factors often improves or cures the problem.

	Corns	Warts
	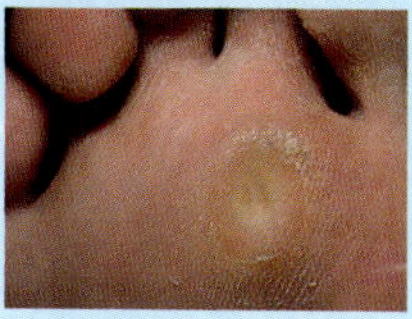	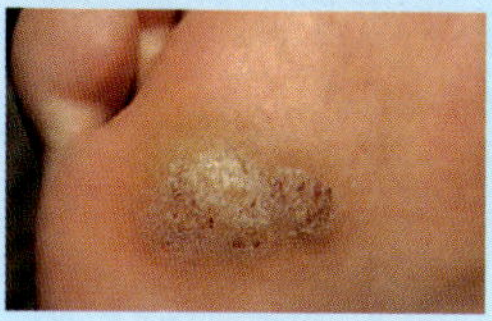
Age	Corns are more common in middle to old age	Plantar warts are more common in children and teenagers
Site	Corns occur almost exclusively on areas subject to pressure	Plantar warts may occur on any part of the foot
Pain	Corns hurt on direct pressure to the lesion	Plantar warts hurt more when pinched
Appearance	Corns, on close examination, will show continuation of normal dermatoglyphics over the lesion	Plantar warts have no continuation of dermatoglyphics over the lesions
Course	Corns will usually only resolve when the causative pressure is relieved	Plantar warts may resolve spontaneously

Table 10
Differential diagnosis between a corn and a verruca (plantar wart)

Hallux abductovalgus

Hallux abductovalgus is a progressive deviation of the big toe away from the midline of the body, often accompanied by a valgus rotation of the toe (Figure 12). As the big toe deviates, a medial prominence develops on the first metatarsal head and becomes inflamed as it rubs on footwear. The second digit frequently overrides the deviating big toe or develops a hammer deformity. The condition occurs most commonly in women and usually shows a familial pattern. The exact aetiology is unknown – many theories have been postulated. Most frequently poor footwear has been implicated, although studies have shown the existence of hallux abductovalgus in unshod races. Also excessively pronated feet have been highlighted as a predisposing factor; inflammatory joint diseases appear to accelerate its development.

Treatment of the condition depends on the symptoms, primary care being direct relief of discomfort. Altered foot shape can give rise to secondary pressure lesions such as corns and callosities, and prevention of these may be afforded by careful footwear selection and cushioning insoles. Where excessive pronation coexists, the use of orthoses may give relief of symptoms. Surgery for hallux valgus is indicated where severe deformity develops early on or when pain relief is not achieved with conservative methods. The effectiveness of night splints to straighten the big toe is questionable.

Hallux limitus and rigidus

Hallux limitus and rigidus (Figure 13) are common conditions of the first toe where there is either reduced or total loss of dorsiflexion at the metatarsophalangeal joint. The deformity is often accompanied by dorsal enlargement of the first metatarsal head and hyperextension of the big toe. Clinically, the patient is most frequently a man who complains of pain in the morning which often wears off during the day, and is

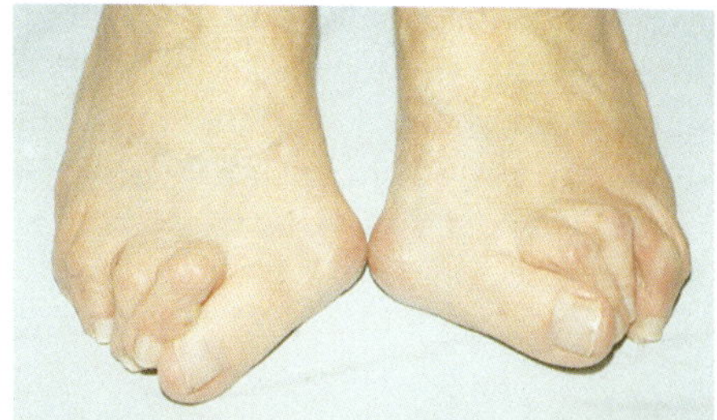

Figure 12
Hallux abductovalgus: rotation of the digit places extra pressure around the nail.

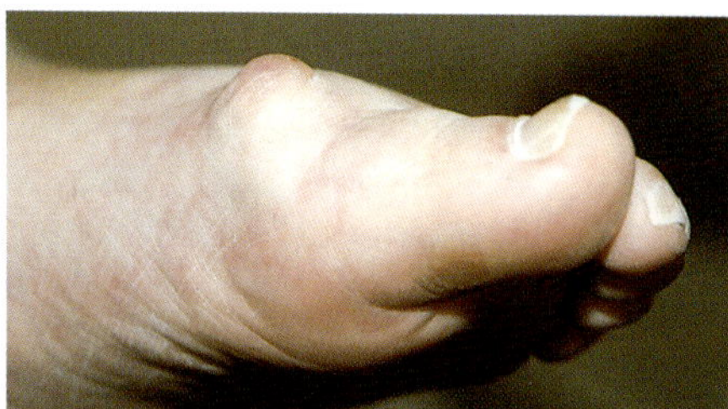

Figure 13
Hallux limitus or rigidus.

aggravated by prolonged standing or activity. Alteration of the normal gait pattern to alleviate the pain may often result in secondary lesions such as plantar corns and callosities, and thickening of the big toe nail.

In normal function the range of motion of the first metatarsophalangeal joint should be sufficient for heel lift and toe dorsiflexion. If this is limited, body weight is forced through the interphalangeal joint of the big toe resulting in hyperextension of the toe and hypertrophy of the nail, leaving them prone to damage from shallow footwear. The primary cause of the disorder is unknown but theories include trauma setting up a localized osteoarthritis in the joint, a long first metatarsal or an excessively pronated foot type causing restriction of normal movement of the foot.

Treatment of the condition is by symptomatic relief. Elimination of aggravating factors may help, i.e. footwear modification/ advice. Insoles and orthoses are of benefit to realign the foot and redistribute weight-bearing away from the painful joint. In acute stages of the disease, immobilization, by way of strapping of the toe, may be of benefit.

Lesser toe deformities

These can be congenital or acquired. The stability and function of the digit is easily altered by abnormal foot function (excessive pronation and supination)(Table 11).

Congenital:

Syndactyly

Spina bifida

Acquired:

Abnormal foot function
e.g. excessive pronation and supination

Poorly fitting footwear
e.g. high heels, lack of fastening, constrictive toe box

Trauma

Inflammatory joint disease
e.g. rheumatoid arthritis, gout, etc.

Neurological diseases
e.g. flaccid and spastic paralysis

Intrinsic foot muscle imbalances

Idiopathic

Table 11
Common causes of digital deformity

Figure 14 outlines some of the more common digital deformities:

- Clawing or retraction of toes arises most commonly as the result of inflammatory joint disease or supinated foot types. Plantarflexion of the metatarsals gives a mechanical advantage to the long extensor tendons of the foot, which inevitably pull the toes into dorsal retraction. Consequently, this causes rubbing on footwear and hyperkeratoses develop on the toes. Moreover, excessive weight is borne on the now prominent metatarsal heads, because digital weight-bearing is diminished, and this leads to metatarsalgia.

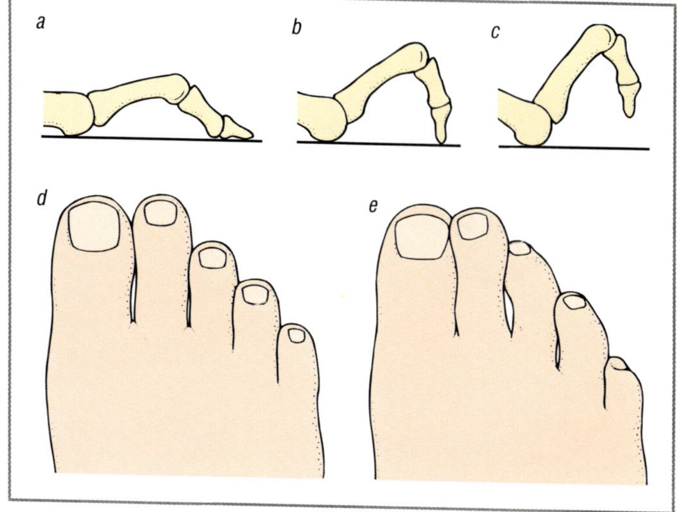

Figure 14
Common digital deformities:
a) Hammer toe
b) Clawed toe (apex of digit in ground contact)
c) Retracted toe (apex not in ground contact)
d) Normal digital alignment
e) Adductovarus deformity of fifth, fourth and third digits

- Adductovarus deformity of the lesser toes is thought to be a result of excessive pronation, flattening the arch and altering the angle of pull of the long flexor tendons. Hyperkeratotic lesions are common on the apices of these toes.
- Hammer toe deformity is often a secondary effect seen with hallux abductovalgus; rarely is it a congenital deformity (Figure 15, and see Figure 14).

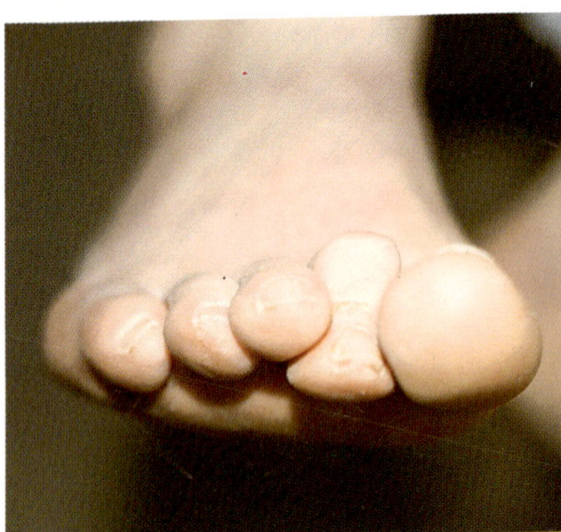

Figure 15
Hammer toe.

Treatment of digital deformities

Where hyperkeratoses have developed on deformed digits, débridement of the lesions may give temporary relief; however, prevention of their recurrence is essential. Footwear must fit correctly if further problems are to be avoided. Podiatrists often use silicon or felt toe props (Figures 16 and 17) to offload high pressure from the affected digits. Surgical arthrodesis or arthroplasty of the lesser toes is often performed to correct the deformity.

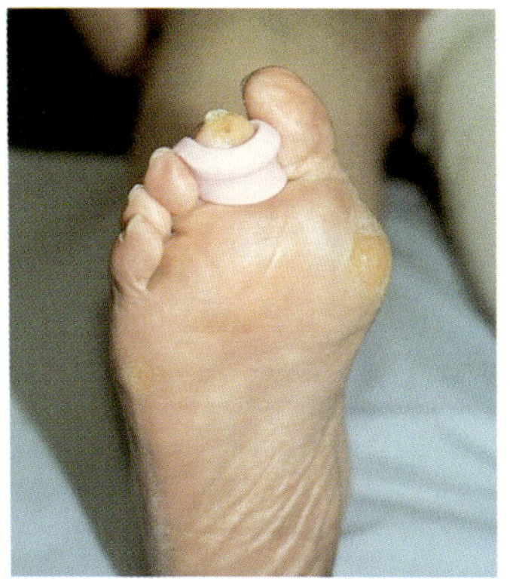

Figure 16
Silicon toe prop – designed to prevent apical weight-bearing in deformed toes.

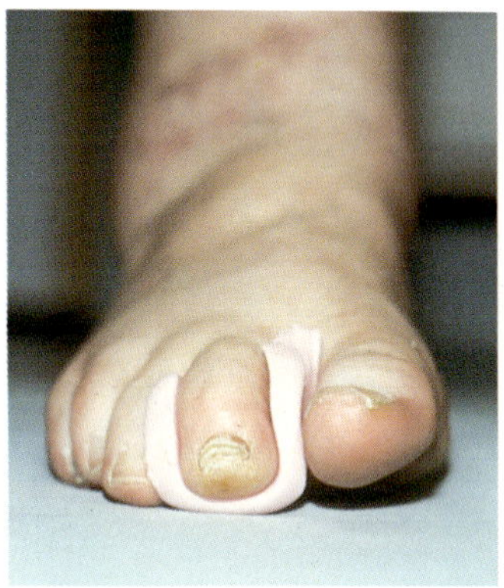

Figure 17
Same silicon toe prop as shown in Figure 16.

Nail changes

Nail deformity often occurs as an end result of digital deformity compounded by poorly fitting footwear, of trauma, or of altered foot shape resulting from other problems such as hallux abductovalgus (see Figure 12).

Subungual haematoma

This common condition occurs as the result of acute trauma to the nail plate from injury, poorly fitting footwear or after long-distance running (e.g. marathon races) (Figures 18 and 19). Haemorrhage leads to the accumulation of blood under the nail plate, forcing its separation from the nail bed which causes pain. Prompt release of the haematoma (within 24 hours) by piercing the nail plate improves the chances of retaining the nail and affords pain relief. Lesions resembling a subungual haematoma without a history of trauma should be monitored and regarded with suspicion because, rarely, the condition may mimic subungual melanoma.

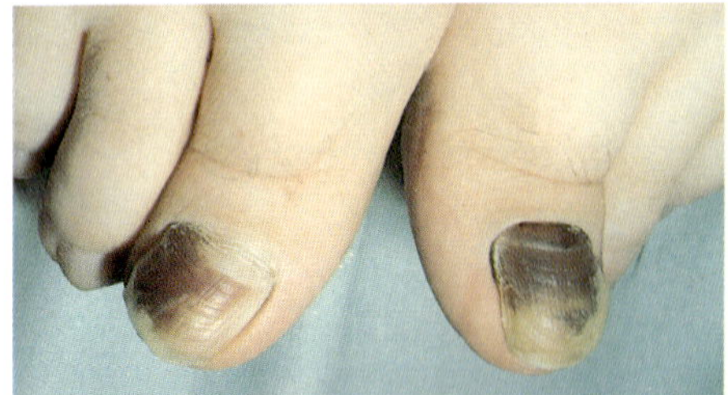

Figure 18
Subungual haematoma.

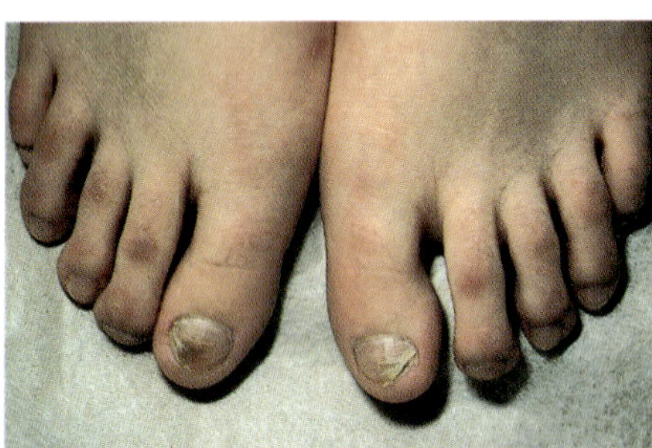

Figure 19
Subungual haematoma, traumatic onycholysis and dorsal corns – long-distance runner.

Onychauxis and onychogryphosis

Onychauxis is a thickening of the entire nail plate (Figure 20). Most commonly observed in the big toe, the condition is often the result of trauma (repeated or single) to the nail although skin disease, such as psoriasis, may also lead to the condition. Digital deformity can accompany the condition. It is more commonly seen in elderly people, and a fungal nail infection may infiltrate the nail.

Onychogryphosis (Figure 21) is a similar affliction, but in this case the nail tends to deviate laterally as it grows. This is usually the result of trauma (occupational or footwear) or sometimes results from earlier untreated onychomycosis. As the nail thickens, nail care becomes difficult. Podiatric treatment of the affected nails is by reduction of the thickened plate with a nail drill. Total avulsion of the nail plate with phenolization of the nail matrix offers a permanent solution to the problem.

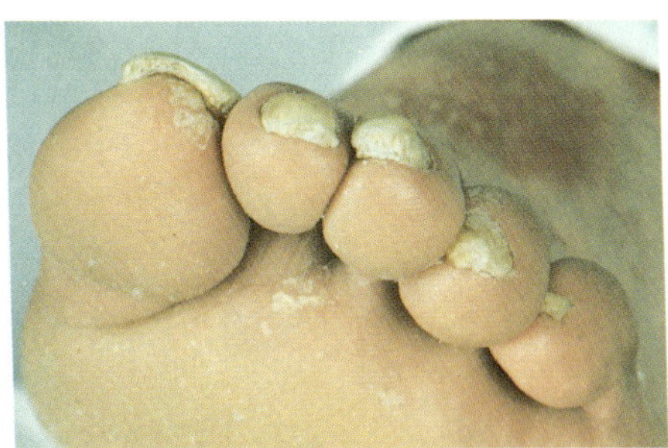

Figure 20
Thickening of nails (onychauxis) as a result of trauma.

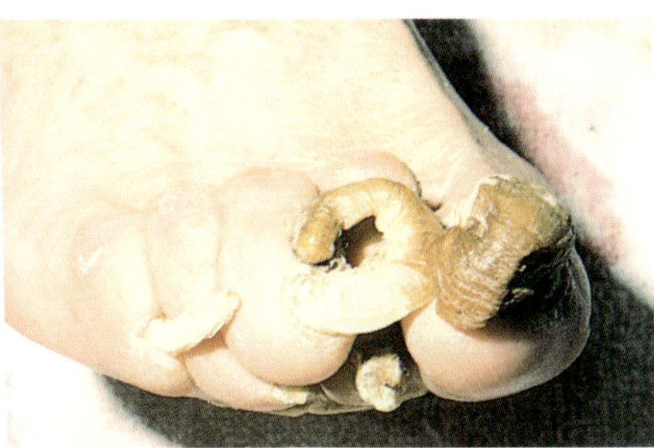

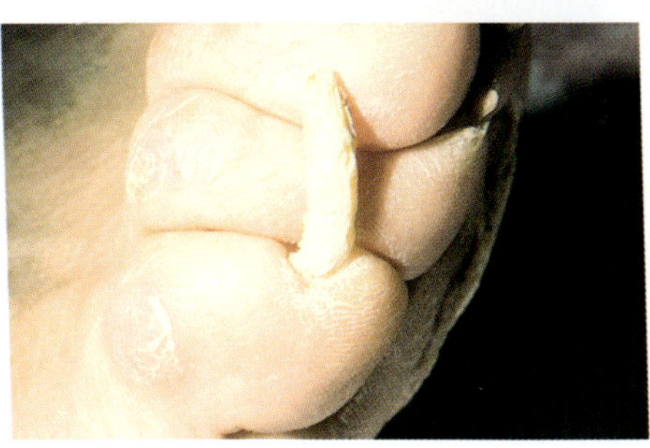

Figure 21
Two examples of onychogryphosis - ram's horn deformity.

Onychocryptosis (ingrowing toe nail)

This is the embedding of the lateral toenail edges into the sulci, piercing the flesh, and leading to local paronychia and secondary bacterial infection.

The condition is most commonly observed in the big toe of physically active young adult men and can result from poor nail cutting technique aggravated by footwear and trauma (Figure 22). Particular nail shapes may be at greater risk of developing the problem. As the embedded nail grows forward, hypergranulation tissue may protrude from the nail sulcus.

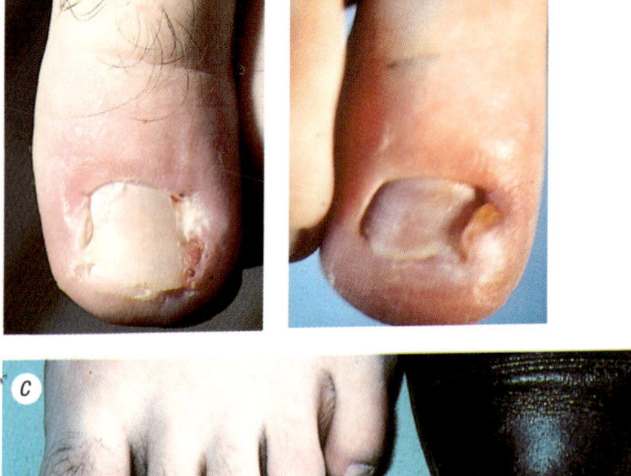

Figure 22
Ingrowing toenail (onychocryptosis): (a) epithelialized; (b) bilateral; and (c) mainly caused by inappropriate footwear.

Isolated occurrences of onychocryptosis may be resolved by conservative removal of the offending spicule and packing the sulcus with cotton wool. Antibiotic cover should be given where secondary bacterial infection is suspected. Education is vital to minimize recurrence. Where the problem is recurrent, lateral nail avulsion, under local anaesthetic with phenolization of the associated matrix, is usually successful (see 'Therapies', page 64).

Local and systemic inflammatory diseases

Inflammatory diseases in the foot produce a classic series of signs: heat (calor), redness (rubor), swelling (tumour), pain (dolor) and loss of function of the affected area, and can involve any of the tissues within the foot (see 'Anatomy of the foot and nail', page 1). The presence of inflammation may be associated with a raised erythrocyte sedimentation rate (ESR). Inflammation can be either superficial or deep (Table 12). A good knowledge of anatomy will help with identification of the site of deep inflammation, and thus aid diagnosis. General causes of inflammation are given in Table 13.

Severe skin inflammation and cellulitis are seen with bacterial infections, but viral and fungal infections usually cause moderate amounts of localized inflammation (see later).

Superficial inflammation

Presentation:	Obvious swelling Tissues warm/hot Tissues red/dusky Patient complains of pain
Examples of causes of superficial inflammation:	
Bacterial infections	Boils, acute paronychia (Figure 23), cellulitis, ingrowing toenail (see 'Therapies', page 64) 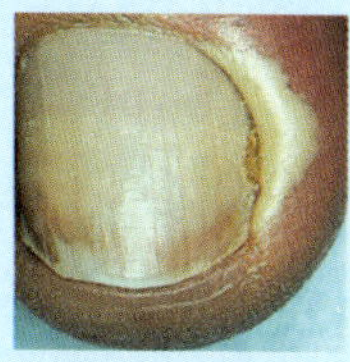 ***Figure 23*** *Acute, purulent inflammatory signs in acute bacterial paronychia.*
Viral infections	Verrucae, molluscum contagiosum (see 'Infective diseases', page 53)
Fungal infections	Yeasts and dermatophytes – athlete's foot (see 'Infective diseases', page 53)
Dermatitis	Atopic, irritant or allergic types (Figures 24 and 25) 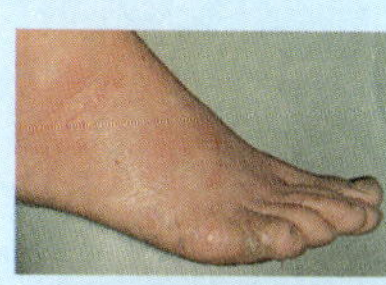 ***Figure 24*** *Allergic dermatitis of the foot.* 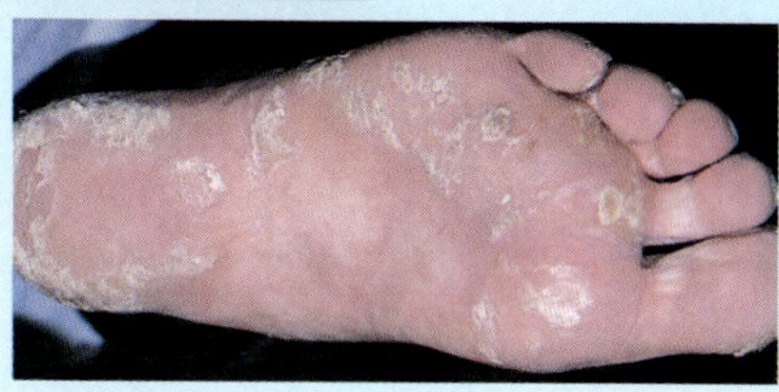 ***Figure 25*** *Chronic constitutional dermatitis of the sole of the foot.*
Psoriasis	Plaque, pustular and nail types (Figures 26 and 27)

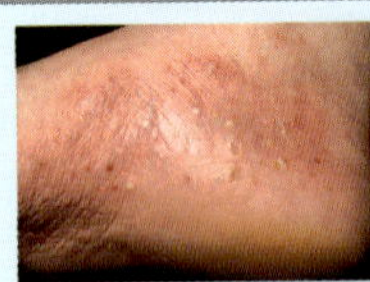

Figure 26
Pustular psoriasis of the foot.

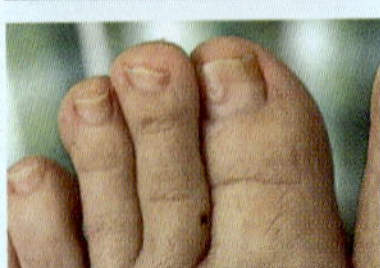

Figure 27
Psoriasis of the nails with some pustulation.

Hypersensitivity reactions	Hives, bites, stings
Acantholysis	Blisters, pemphigus
Ulcers and breakdowns	Ischaemia, neuropathy, rheumatoid diseases, trauma; corn plasters; thermal injury

Deep inflammation

Presentation:	Patient complains of pain, especially on movement Movement difficult Pain elicited by palpation of the particular site Warmth Possible oedema
Examples of causes of deep inflammation:	
Bursitis	Of both congenital and adventitious bursae
Panniculitis	Of the plantar fibrofatty pad
Foot strain Plantar fasciitis Heel spur	Especially with excess subtalar joint and midtarsal pronation
Arthritis/arthrosis	In rheumatoid arthritis, osteoarthritis, gout
Osteomyelitis	Bone infection from a deep perforating ulcer, or as a blood-borne infection from a more central site

Table 12
Superficial and deep inflammation

Causes	Inflammation
Mechanical injury	Overpronation at STJ/MTJ; strains, sprains, fractures, osteoarthrosis, blisters, corns and callosities
Thermal injury	Cryosurgery, chilblain, Raynaud's disease, electrosurgery and cauterisation; burns; sunburn
Chemical injury	Corn plasters, acids, release of histamine in hypersensitivity reaction (allergy, atopy, bites, stings)
Infection	Bacteria, fungi, viruses
Autoimmunity	Rheumatoid diseases

Table 13
Causes of inflammation

Specific examples of inflammatory pathologies in the foot

Bursae

Congenital bursae are found normally in the foot, but adventitious bursae may form as a synovial sac in superficial tissues, in response to ongoing shear stresses. Additional stress can cause inflammation of the sac – bursitis. Inflamed bursae may perforate or ulcerate, and undergo bacterial infection. Patients with rheumatoid diseases may have large, inflamed and swollen bursae overlying the plantar aspects of the metatarsal heads. Common sites for bursae are shown in Figure 28.

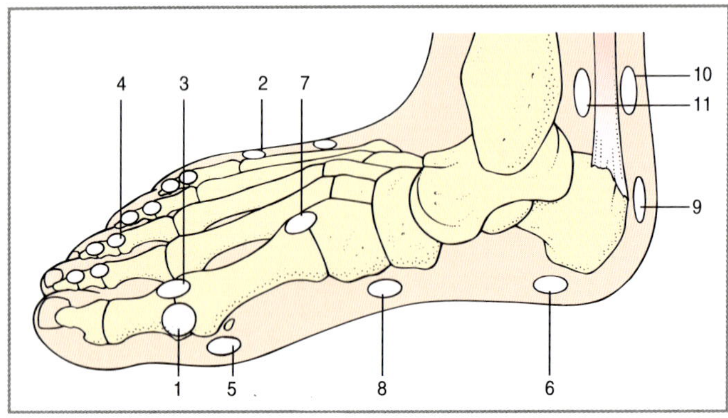

Figure 28
Common sites of bursae in the foot:

1 *Medial side of the 1 MTPJ, in hallux abductovalgus, forming a 'bunion'*
2 *Lateral side of the 5 MTPJ in hallux abductovalgus, forming a tailor's bunion, or 'bunionette'*
3 *Dorsum of the 1 MTPJ, in hallux rigidus, or late stage osteoarthritis of the joint*
4 *Dorsa of the lesser toes, in clawed, hammered, retracted or otherwise deformed toes, often complicated by overlying corn formation*
5 *Plantar aspect of the MTPJs, in rheumatoid patients, with ulceration*
6 *Plantar aspect of the heel — 'policeman's heel' seen in subjects who have to stand about a great deal, or subjects who are obese,or those who have pes cavus*
7 *Dorsal aspect of the tarsus (midfoot) in subjects with pes cavus*
8 *Plantar aspect of the tarsal area of the medial longitudinal arch in subjects with flat foot; this may ulcerate in neuropathic or ischaemic subjects*
9 *Retrocalcaneal area, especially in subjects who overpronate, where the heel counter rubs against the lateroposterior area of the heel; this area often is subject to blistering, and may form additional bumps of bone (pump bumps/Haglund's deformity)*
10 *Superficial to Achilles tendon, especially where the heel counter is very curved and traumatizes the soft tissues, or in pes cavus/functional ankle equinus*
11 *Deep to Achilles tendon forming swollen areas either side, just above the heel*

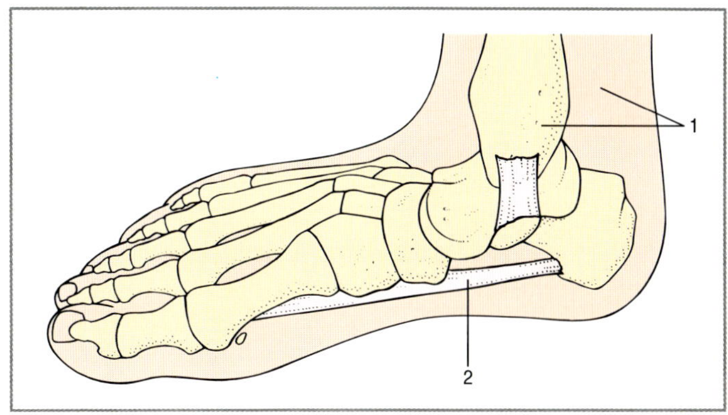

Figure 29
Common sites of pain associated with ligamentous strain and sprains in the foot:

1 *Patients with pes cavus are subject to repeated lateral ankle sprains; Flat-footed subjects are subject to medial ankle sprains, and painful pinching of the lateral soft tissues below the lateral malleolus*

2 *The deep plantar fasciae are subject to chronic overstretching in subjects with hypermobile feet, and in those with excess pronation at the STJ and MTJ, causing foot strain or plantar fasciitis*
The patient complains of low-grade pain and a perpetual tiredness in the feet, especially the medial longitudinal arch
Commonly the heel area is very tender, especially over the plantar medial tubercle of the calcaneum

Strains and sprains

The more fibrous the tissue, the less vascular it is likely to be. Fibrous structures such as the plantar fascia rarely become acutely inflamed, but as a result of their relatively avascular nature they take longer to undergo a process of repair. Ligaments are vulnerable to further injury during the healing time. Deep ligament tears are accompanied by a great deal of local soft-tissue damage. The most common sites for pain experienced with sprains are shown in Figure 29.

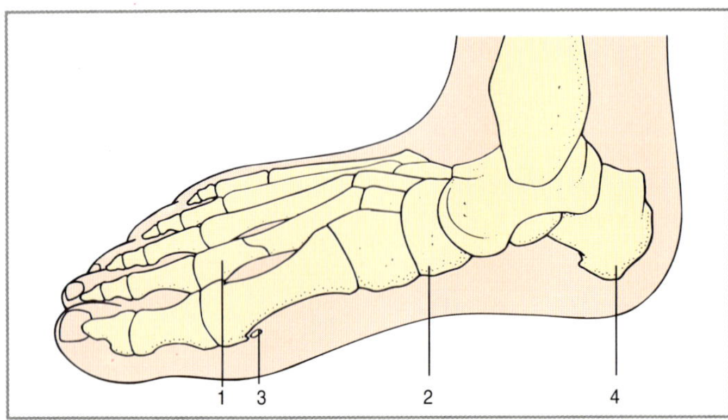

Figure 30
Effect of inflammation in bone

- *Late stage inflammatory arthritides show new bone formation (osteophytes) at the margins of affected joints.*
- *Enthesiopathy: tension at the insertion of the plantar fascia causes lifting of the periosteum, and formation of a heel spur.*
- *Chronic mechanical stress can cause march fracture in metatarsals, or a plantar-flexed 1st metatarsal can lead to stress fracture of a sesamoid.*
- *Neuropathic joint foot surfaces undergo microfracture, and development of Charcot's arthropathy.*
- *Avascular necrosis causes an area of cancellous bone to become ischaemic and die. The surrounding healthy bone collapses in, causing flattening of the (1) 2nd metatarsal head (Freiberg's disease), (2) navicular bone (Kohler's disease), (3) medial sesamoid bone (Kohler's second disease), (4) posterior surface of the heels (Sever's disease). Children are most commonly affected.*

Effects of inflammation at bone surfaces

The effects of inflammation in bone are shown in Figure 30.

Inflammation in tendons

The synovial sheaths of the extrinsic tendons may undergo a process of inflammation – tendonitis – as a result of chronic overuse or sudden twisting trauma, or in rheumatoid diseases. The problems that can arise are illustrated in Figure 31.

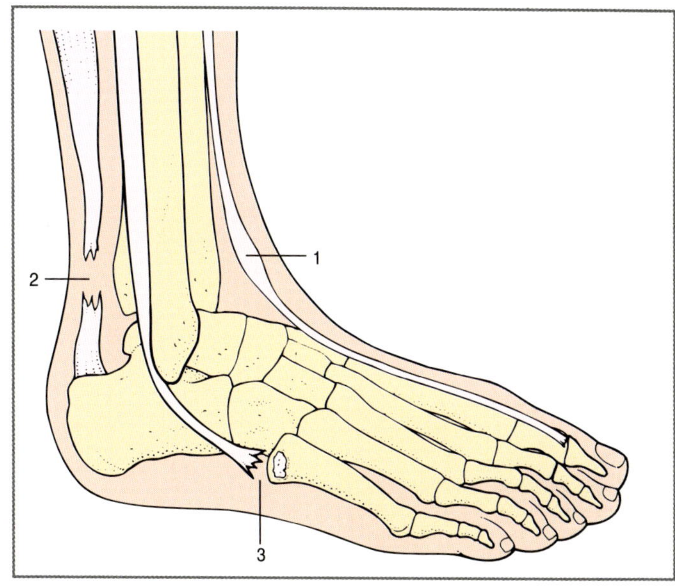

Figure 31
Inflammatory tendon problems are associated with:
1 *Rheumatoid arthritis – tendonitis*
2 *Sudden, unaccustomed movements, especially in patients who have undertaken sudden exercise – full or partial rupture of Achilles tendon*
3 *Growing adolescents (12-14 year old girls) – avulsion of a tuberosity at tendon insertion (insertion of peroneus tertius into the base of the 5th metatarsal)*

Inflammatory joint diseases

Joint pathologies are characterized by inflammation and include: the seropositive arthritides, e.g. rheumatoid arthritis; seronegative arthritides, e.g. osteoarthritis and chronic hallux ridigus; metabolic arthropathies, e.g. gout; infective arthropathies, e.g. rubellar arthritis, tubercular arthritis, Reiter's disease; and mechanical arthritides, e.g. acute hallux limitus, hallux valgus. Characteristics and symptoms of inflammatory joint diseases are shown in Tables 14 and 15 and Figure 32.

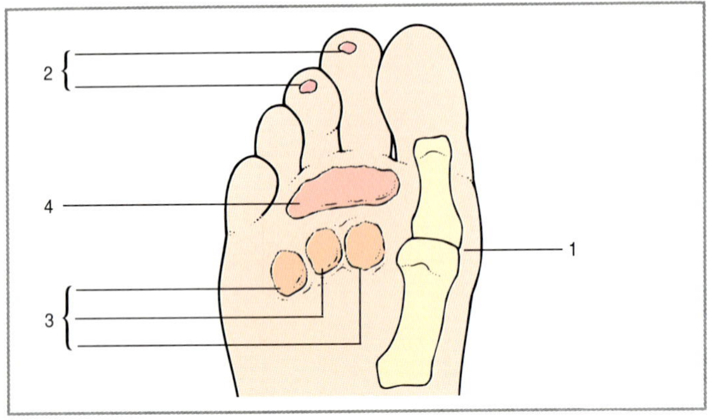

Figure 32
Soft tissue symptoms of inflammatory joint disease in the foot:

1 *Gouty tophi*
Deposition of insoluble sodium urate crystal within joint tissues causes a profound acute inflammatory reaction. Similarly, urate may be deposited in non-articular soft tissues, such as overlying a lesser toe joint, or subungually. The overlying soft tissues ulcerate, and urate leaches from the ulcer, as a bright, white granular discharge. The ulcer will not heal until all the urate is removed from the area, and the underlying gouty process is controlled by medication

2 *Vasculitis (Figures 33—35)*
Blood-borne immune complexes block distal capillaries, causing tiny areas of thrombosis, in the form of pin-point patches of skin necrosis. Where these occur subungually, they appear as fine 'splinter' haemorrhages (Figure 36); where a number of vasculitic areas are close together, the skin may ulcerate. Vasculitic episodes are also seen with sickle cell anaemia, where abnormal erythrocytes will clump together, blocking arterioles and capillaries, especially in conditions of low oxygen tension or under the stimulus of cold

3 *Rheumatoid bursae*
Acutely painful, enlarged and distended bursae form on the plantar aspect of the metatarsophalangeal joints. The skin overlying them is subject to callous formation; a sinus may develop the area may ulcerate.

4 *Panniculitis*
Chronic inflammation of the weight-bearing plantar fibrofatty tissues, the plantar fibrofatty pad is drawn distally where the lesser toes are clawed, retracted or distorted, becomes pinched and traumatized, and exposes the MTPJs to ground reaction forces.

Figure 33
Purpuric vasculitis.

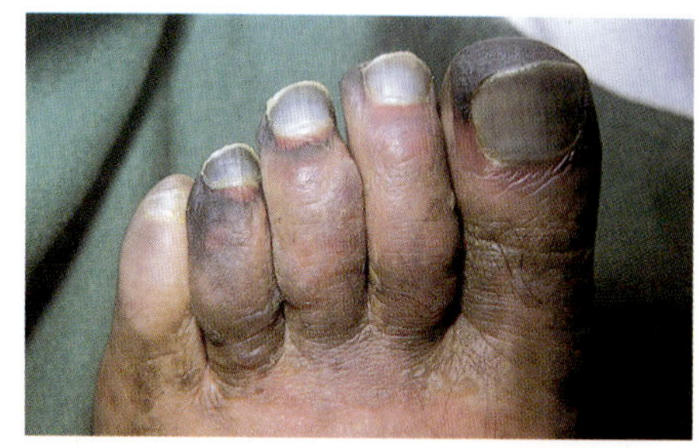

Figure 34
Streptococcal vasculitis.

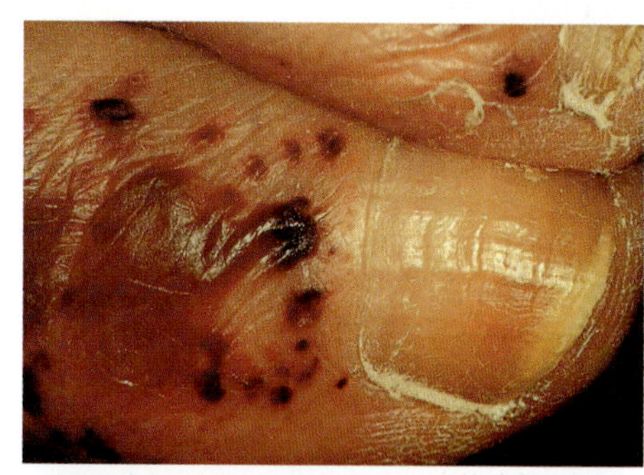

Figure 35
Vascular inflammation and necrosis due to systemic sclerosis.

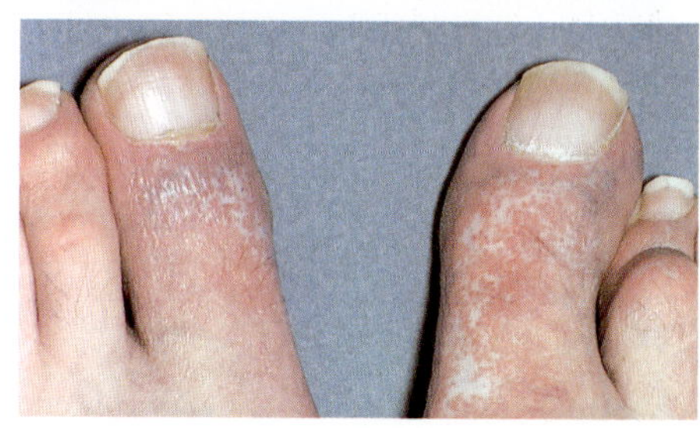

Figure 36
Splinter haemorrhages under the nail.

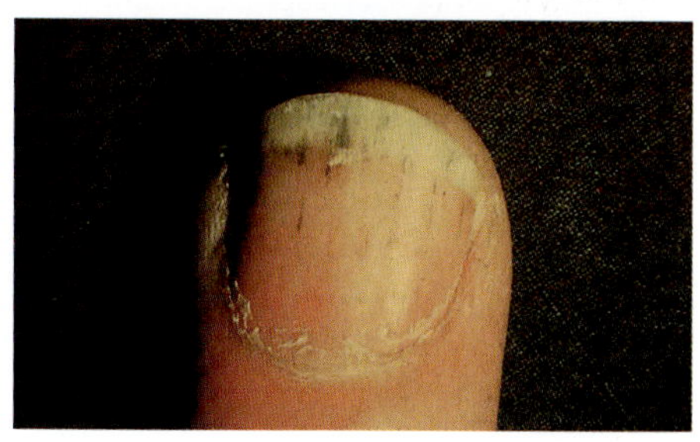

Seropositive arthritis, e.g. rheumatoid arthritis; juvenile chronic arthritis (Still's disease); CREST diseases

Characteristic pattern of joint deterioration, over a period of years:

- initial swelling and proliferation of the synovial lining of the joint erosion of joint surfaces
- cystic degeneration of bone
- presence of rheumatoid factor in blood

Affected joints:

- initially hot, red, swollen and tender
- movement hampered by pain and stiffness, especially in the morning
- 5 MTPJ is often the first foot joint affected.

Large plantar bursae develop over the MTPJs

Gross joint deformity (of the 1 and 5 MTPJs, and STJ) with subluxation

Nerve entrapment at the ankle:

- Tinel's sign (paraesthesiae) of the sole of the foot.

Other serious systemic effects:

- heart, lung and kidney problems, keratoconjunctivitis sicca

Seronegative arthritides, e.g. osteoarthritis; some forms of rheumatoid arthritis and ankylosing spondylitis

Characteristic pattern of joint deterioration:

- gradual loss of integrity of the articular cartilage
- development of osteophytic outgrowths from bone edges
- limitation of joint movement and local swelling
- late stage joint ankylosis

Affects the major weight-bearing joints:

- hip
- knee
- 1 MTPJ, as the end stage of hallux limitus / rigidus

Metabolic arthropathy, e.g. gout, pseudogout

Urate crystals are deposited in the 1 MTPJ, causing an acute arthritis

- the joint becomes very inflamed, usually over the course of a night
- gross swelling and redness
- exquisite tenderness
- attack subsides in a few days

In the long term, subjects usually develop osteoarthritis at the affected joint

Urates are deposited in soft tissues causing formation of gouty tophi:

- pinna of the ear
- subungually
- dorsum of lesser toe joints

Infective arthritis

Arises as:

- local spread of infection from a bacterial infection of a bursa (infected bursitis) or bone (osteomyelitis)

Systemic viral infections (rubella, or enterococcal infections)

- temporary arthritis affecting the small joints

E. coli infections

- generalized arthropathy, as part of Reiter's disease

Table 14
Characteristics of inflammatory joint disease

Seropositive (e.g. rheumatoid arthritis)	Seronegative (e.g. osteoarthritis)
Generalized systemic disease affecting all connective tissues, including joints	Generalized joint disease, or localized joint disease
Initially affects children and young/middle-aged adults	May affect young people — as the result of isolated traumatic episode Generally affects elderly people
Attacks small joints of the hands and feet, especially 1 and 5 MTPJs	Attacks large weight-bearing joints: hip, knee, 1 MTPJ
Causes pannus formation (proliferation of the synovial membrane), obliterating cartilage and causing periarticular erosions and subluxation of the joint	Causes exposure and fibrillation of cartilage, and eburnation of exposed bone, loss of articular space, osteophyte formation, sclerosis, cystic degeneration, limitation of movement and eventual ankylosis of the joint
Is especially painful in the morning	It is usually painful on movement, but may cease when the affected joint has become ankylosed

Table 15
Characteristics of seropositive and seronegative arthritides

Ulceration

The various types of ulcer seen in the foot are given in Table 16, and the typical sites of occurrence are shown in Figure 37.

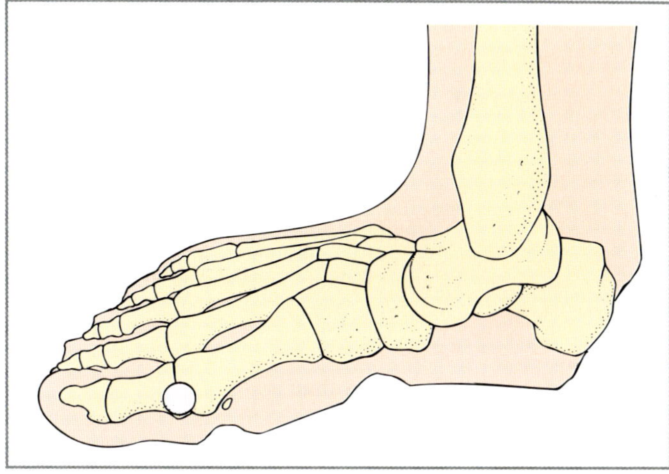

Figure 37
Typical sites for foot ulceration

- *Bony prominences including:*
  - *Medial aspect of 1 MTPJ*
  - *Lateral side of the tuberosity at the base of the 5th metatarsal*
  - *The plantar aspect of the MTPJs*
  - *The interdigital skin overlying the proximal and distal interphalangeal joints*
  - *The dorsal skin overlying the proximal and distal interphalangeal joints*
- *The medial longitudinal arch, in*
  - *pes planus*
  - *Charcot's arthropathy of the tarsal area*
- *The posterior/inferior angle of the heel, with prolonged bed rest*
- *The tips of the toes, and bony prominences with:*
  - *Generalized ischaemia*
  - *Raynaud's disease*
  - *Chilling*
- *Subungual tissues, with:*
  - *Onychauxis*
  - *Onychogryphosis*
  - *Subungual haematoma*
  - *Subungual gouty tophi*

Trophic (neuropathic) ulcer

Seen with diabetes mellitus (Figure 38) and Hansen's disease

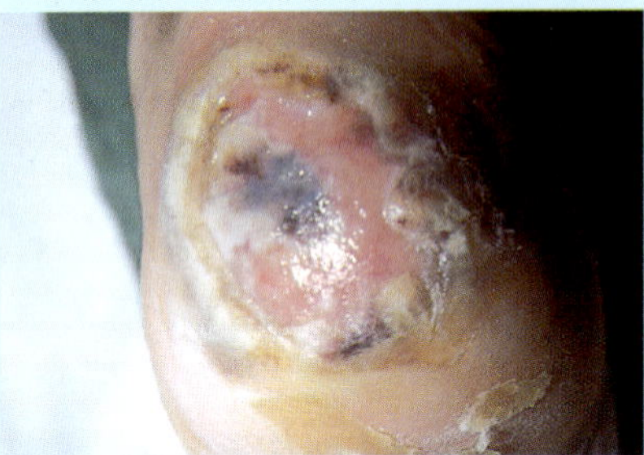

Figure 38
Diabetic heel: neuropathic, microarteriopathic and pressure ulcer.

Either: Foot assumes a 'claw' shape – traumatization of the skin overlying the metatarsal heads and dorsa of the interphalangeal joints

Or: Tarsal joints develop Charcot's neuroarthopathy

Loss of the medial arch

Abnormal weight-bearing

Vasculitic ulcer

Seen with rheumatoid arthritis, with gross distortion of the joints, especially the 1 MTPJ and the subtalar joint; development of hallux abductovalgus and pes planus

Ulceration occurs over bony prominences and plantar bursae

Cold injury

Seen with severe chilling, chilblains (Figure 39) and Raynaud's disease (Figure 40)

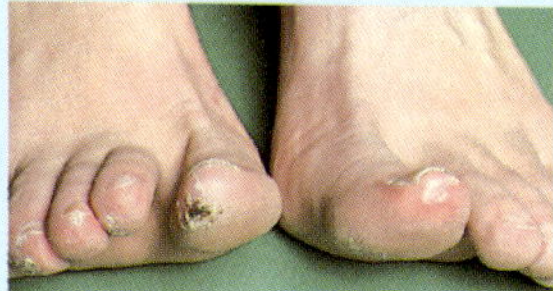

Figure 39
Ulcerated chilblains.

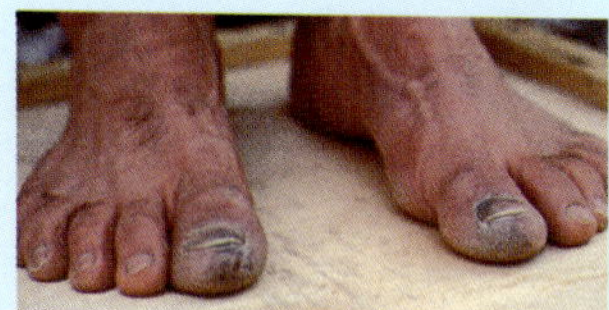

Figure 40
Raynaud's disease: cyanosis and incipient gangrene.

Affected areas of skin undergo a period of ischaemia due to prolonged vasospasm; an acute inflammatory reaction when vessels relax, with resultant blister or bullae formation, or tissue necrosis and ulceration

A similar process occurs in soft tissues overlying bony prominences in patients with generalized foot and limb ischaemia.

Venous ulceration

Venous insufficiency may cause ulceration of the dorsum of the foot

Classic signs of venous incompetence in the lower limb:

oedema
varicose veins
varicose eczema
hemosiderosis
ulceration

Iatrogenic ulceration
Caustic treatments: application of acids to clear corns or verrucae causes tissue destruction; corn paints Thermal treatments of corns or verrucae: cryosurgery; electrosurgery

Malignant ulcers
Malignant melanoma or squamous cell carcinoma may ulcerate – does not usually affect the plantar skin – may involve the nail unit Metastases do not usually invade the foot A long-standing foot ulcer may undergo neoplastic changes (Figure 41)

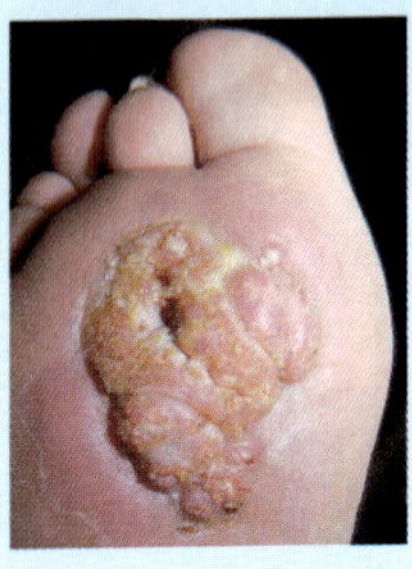

Figure 41
Chronic neuropathic ulcer and squamous carcinoma.

Table 16
Types of ulcer seen in the foot

Infective diseases

Many viral, bacterial and fungal organisms can produce primary or secondary infection of the foot and toenails – or simply colonize other diseases. Note that normal or transient flora may have a job to do – only treat proven pathogens! These normal flora include some staphylococci, corynebacteria, *Pseudomonas* sp (Figure 42) and many fungi of dermatophytic, yeast and saprophytic type.

Bacterial infections

Bacterial infections that may specifically limit themselves to the foot, or cause damage to foot function, include:

- Corynebacteria
  - erythrasma
  - pitted keratolysis
    (synonym, keratolysis plantare sulcatum)
- Streptococci
  - blistering distal dactylitis (Figure 43)
  - erysipelas
- Staphylococci
  - impetigo
  - acute paronychia

- Tuberculosis
  - persistent ulceration
  - warty plaques
  - granulomatous lupus
  - vulgaris plaques
- Leprosy
  - skeletal and skin results of nerve damage

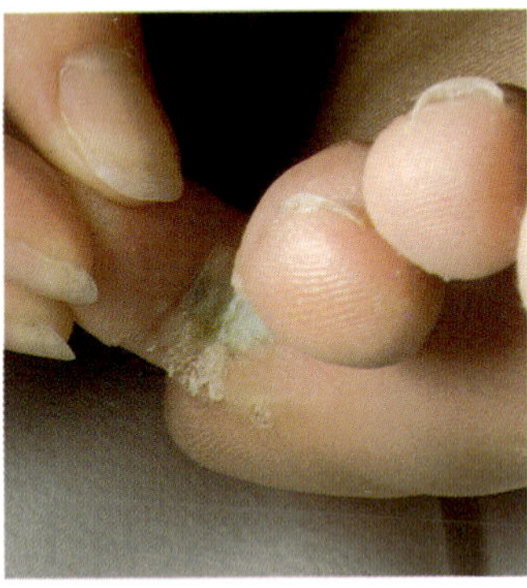

Figure 42
Pseudomonas *sp – green pyocyanin showing in tinea pedis.*

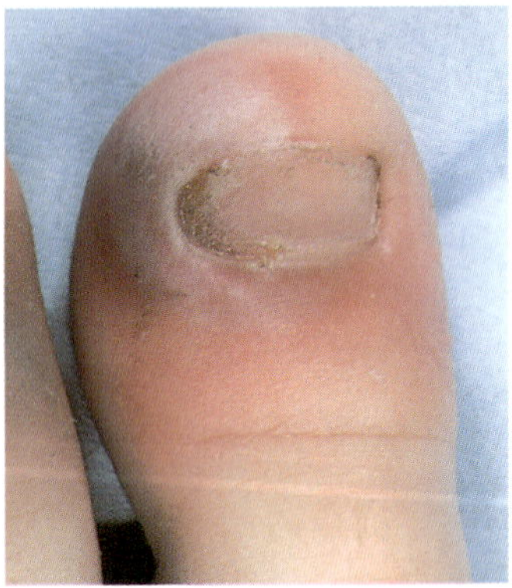

Figure 43
Blistering distal dactylitis – an acute infection caused by haemolytic streptococci.

Pitted keratolysis

As a result of erosion of the keratinous layer of soles of feet by corynebacteria, particularly around sweat pores initially, punctate erosions coalesce to give larger circular lesions. Treatment is of the hyperhidrosis, which is often associated: topical fusidate twice daily for 14 days.

Erythrasma

Coral red fluorescence is seen with Wood's light at sites of colonization – typically third or fourth web space. Various bacteria and dermatophyte fungi may be found concurrently. Treatment is to keep the area dry, plus Whitfield's ointment (3% salicylic acid and 6% benzoic acid), topical fusidate, or oral oxytetracycline.

Viral infections

On the foot, the variety of lesions due to the wart virus, human papilloma virus (HPV), predominate. Though usually no more than an inconvenience, HPV infection may lead to squamous carcinoma, particularly in old and immunosuppressed individuals.

Plantar wart (verruca)

HPV infection commonly occurs on the weight-bearing or pressure parts of the sole or toes; the forefoot is more usually affected than the heel. There may be individual, grouped or mosaic lesions, particularly occurring in older children and young adults – direct infection during barefoot activities (Figures 44–47).

Individual lesions may be asymptomatic and last only a few months. Grouped or mosaic warts may last for years and distort toe or foot function.

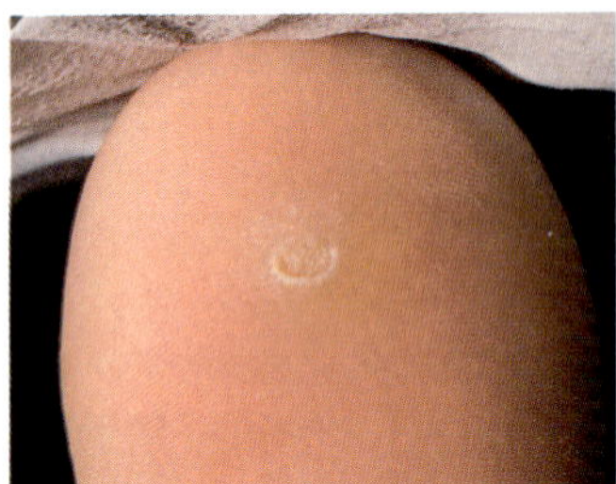

Figure 44
Plantar wart – a single lesion.

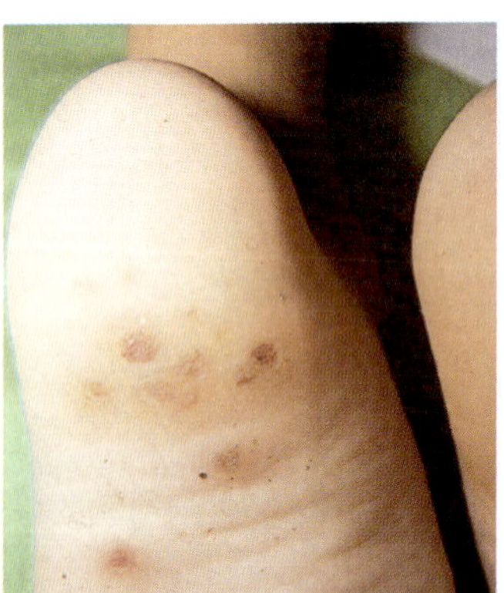

Figure 45
Plantar warts – blackening, resolving lesions.

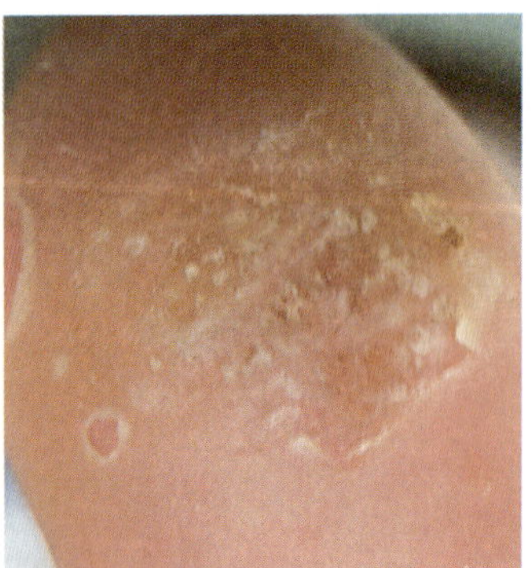

Figure 46
Mosaic plantar wart.

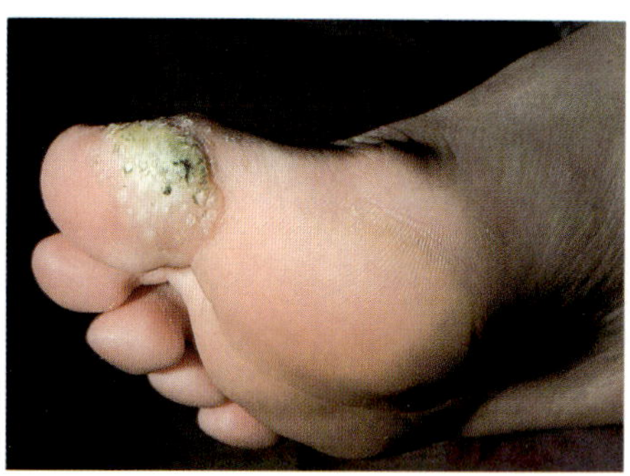

Figure 47
Grouped warts of right great toe.

Periungual warts

These may grow and distort any part of the nail apparatus and persist for many years (Figures 48 and 49). Diagnosis may be difficult – similar to other tumours or swellings such as fibroma (Figure 50), carcinoma in situ (Bowen's disease), squamous carcinoma (Figure 51), or subungual corn (heloma) (Figure 52). Note that 65% remit spontaneously within 2 years.

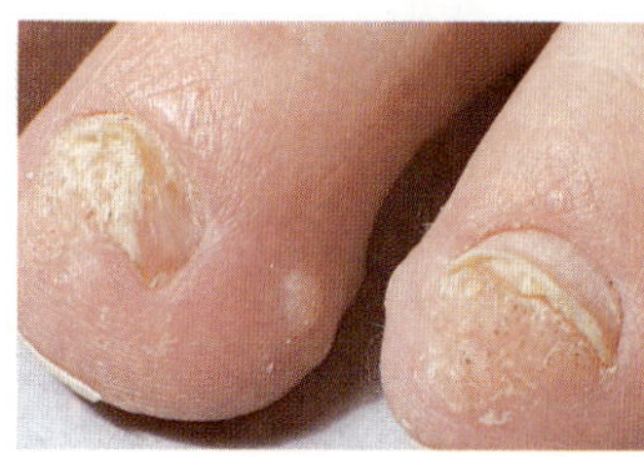

Figure 48
Subungual and periungual warts.

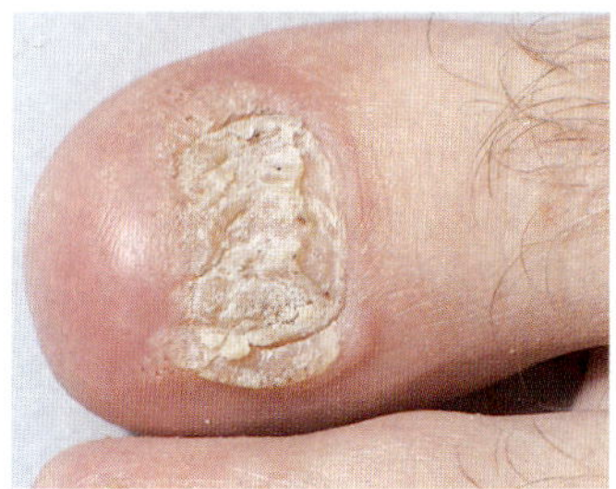

Figure 49
HPV infection invading the whole nail bed, matrix and periungual tissue.

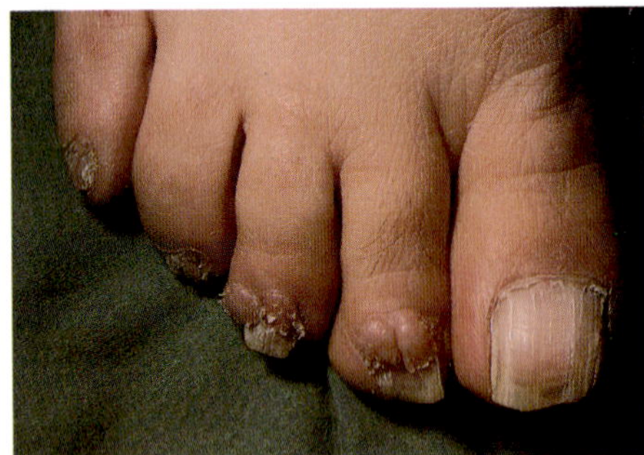

Figure 50
Periungual fibrous (Koenen's) tumours in tuberose sclerosis.

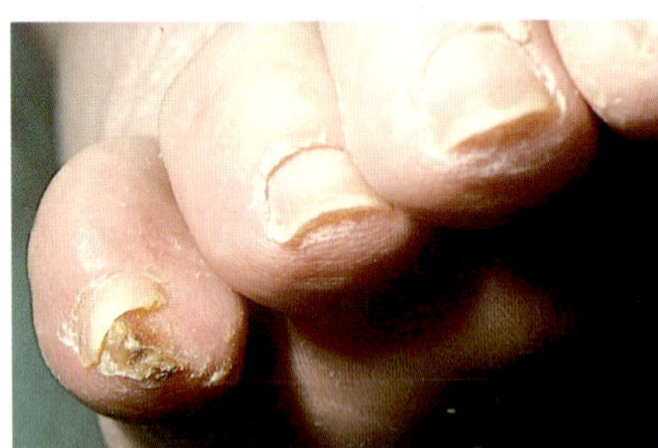

Figure 51
Squamous carcinoma.

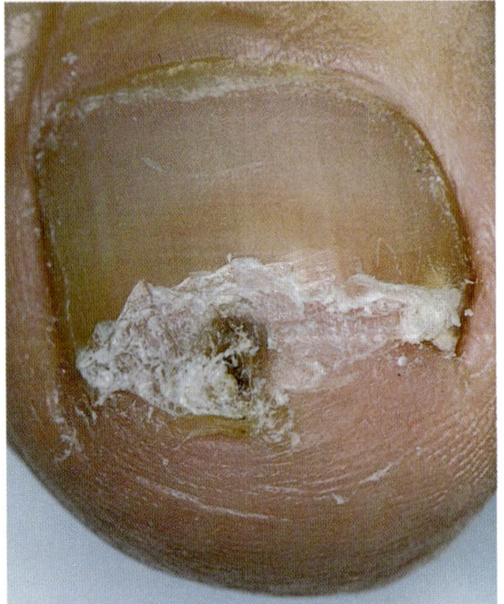

Figure 52
Subungual corn (heloma) – may be painful and haemorrhagic.

Fungal infections

Dermatophytosis

This is a fungal infection of the foot and toenails. At these sites, in clinical practice, dermatophytes are the most common fungi, sometimes saprophytes and rarely yeasts. The genera *Trichophyton* and *Epidermophyton* most frequently cause foot and nail infections, which may be severe or crippling in the immunocompromised.

Infection of the skin, tinea pedis (Figures 53–55), typically starts in the third or fourth web space, with itching, scaling and fissuring. Infection of the sole or dorsum of the foot is rare if the web spaces are normal – under these circumstances, think of other possible causes such as psoriasis (Figure 56) or dermatitis (synonym: eczema).

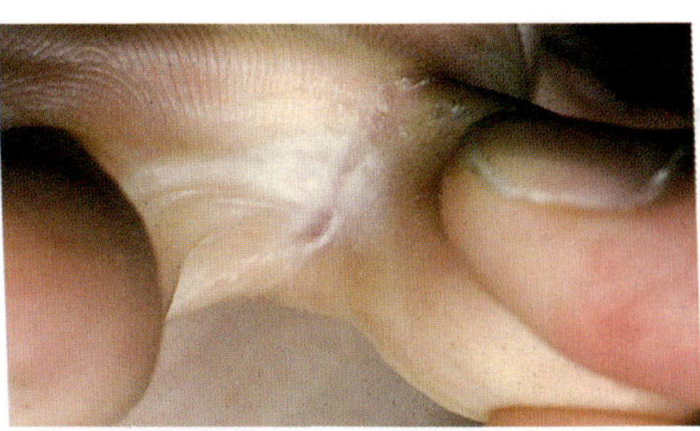

Figure 53
Tinea pedis of web space.

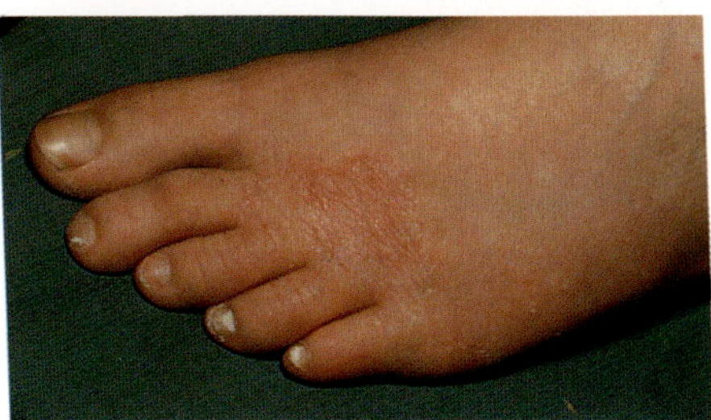

Figure 54
Tinea pedis of dorsum of foot.

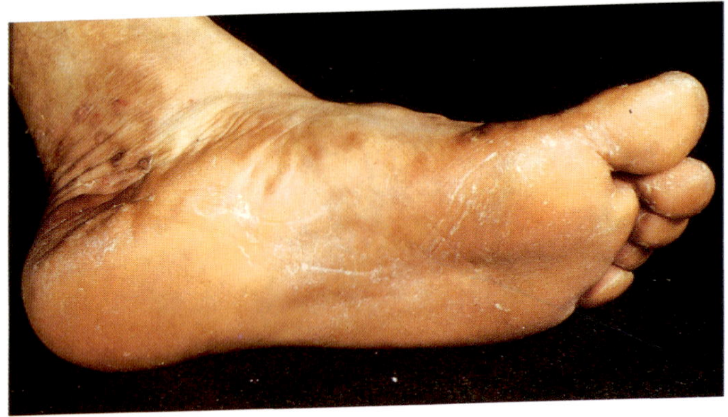

Figure 55
Tinea pedis of sole.

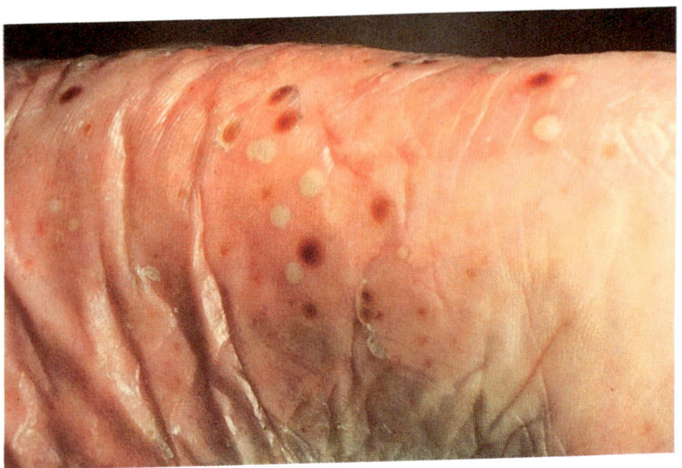

Figure 56
Pustular psoriasis.

Chronic web space infection may be concurrently infected by *Pseudomonas* or *Candida* species. *Trichophyton rubrum* may result in a chronic, asymptomatic, dry and powdery, red appearance of the skin of the foot (Figure 57).

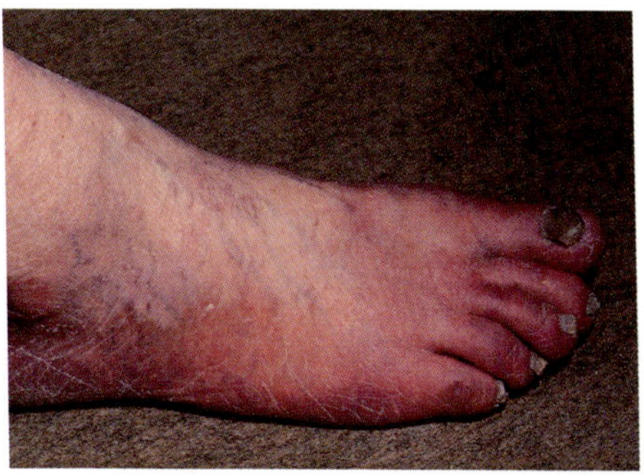

Figure 57
Trichophyton rubrum *infection of the foot and nail.*

Toenail fungal infection, onychomycosis (Figures 58–60), most typically affects the big toenail alone or before other nails. It is usually asymmetrical. Always look at toe and foot function – even minor faults may lead to secondary fungal invasion. This is particularly important when drug treatment fails.

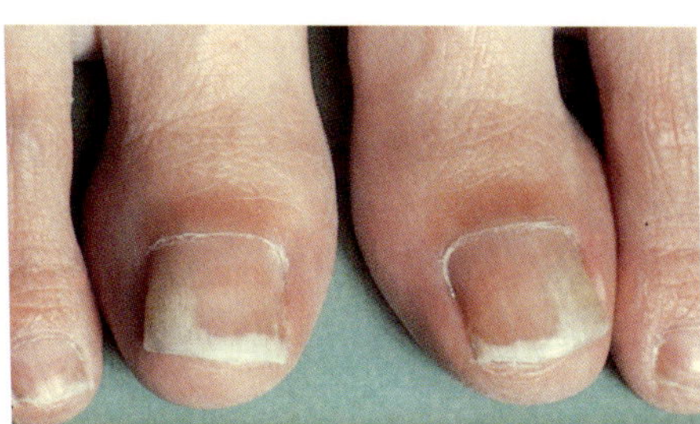

Figure 58
Onychomycosis.

The infection usually starts with distal nail bed invasion, then proximal spread; other entry points are rare (Figure 61). The whole nail bed plate may succumb (Figures 59 and 60). Untreated onychomycosis may lead to ingrowing toenail or onychogryphosis (Figure 60).

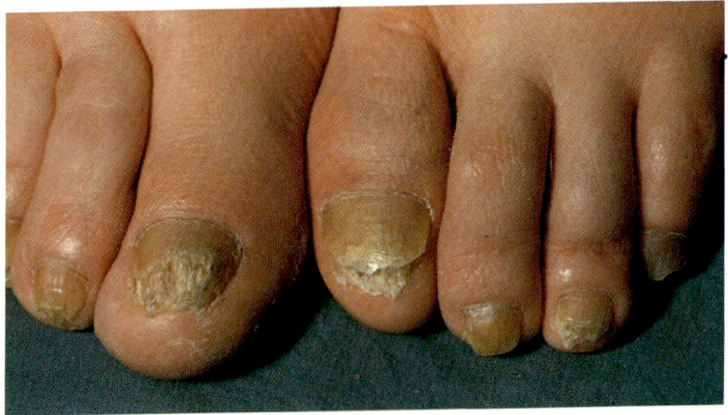

Figure 59
Onychomycosis – total dystrophic type.

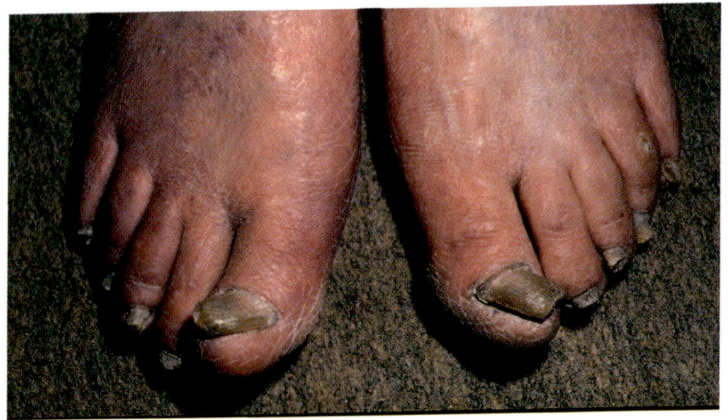

Figure 60
Onychogryphosis due to nail fungal infection (T. rubrum).

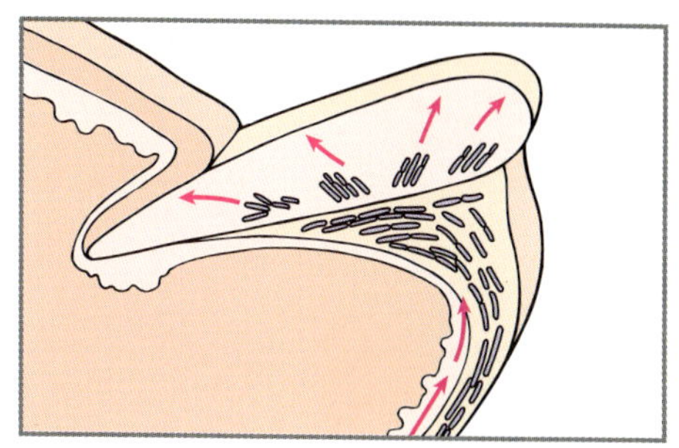

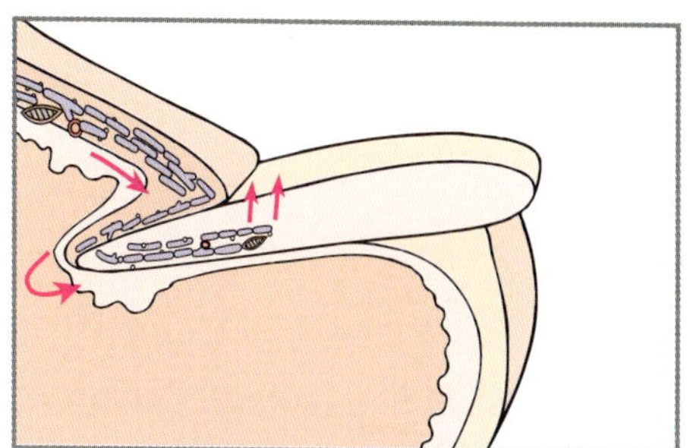

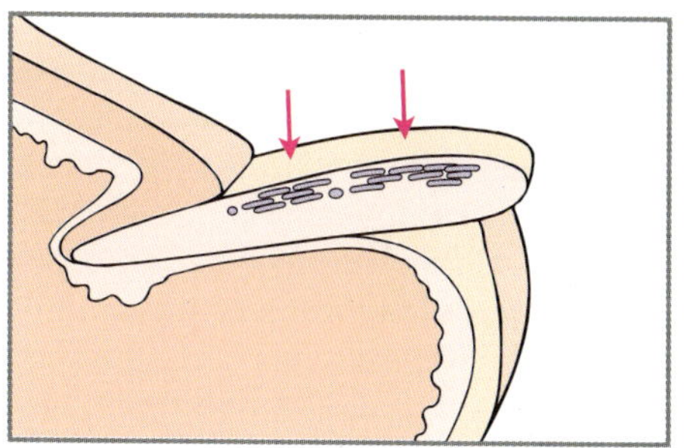

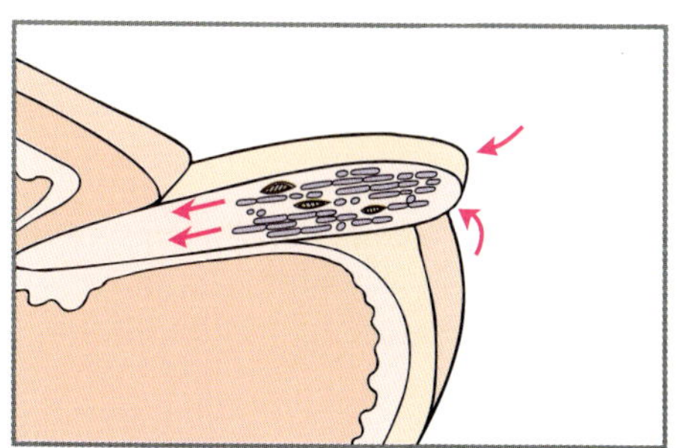

Figure 61
Onychomycosis – arrows show directions of invasion.

Therapies

In this context the specific treatments of tinea pedis, onychomycosis and wart virus infection are considered.

Tinea pedis and onychomycosis

It is important to treat symptomatic tinea pedis and onychomycosis. Untreated tinea pedis may lead to severe reactive inflammation with painful fissuring of the feet and toes. Occasionally, generalized 'autosensitization' eruptions occur in response to persistent focal fungal skin disease. Onychomycosis may be asymptomatic and no more than an 'aesthetic compromise' in its early stages. However, progression of the disease frequently leads to complications such as ingrowing toenail and the painful nail plate deformities of onychogryphosis and pincer or trumpet nail. Studies of onychogryphosis in the elderly show that many such patients had untreated onychomycosis at a younger age. The initial capital cost of successfully treating onychomycosis is therefore fully justified.

On the foot, treatment principles involve either removal of the site of infection, the stratum corneum, with keratolytics or the use of specific antifungal drugs. Rarely, surgical methods may be involved.

Keratolytics may be used alone or in combination with drying or antifungal powders; oral therapy can be used if infection is severe. The most common keratolytic is salicylic acid, e.g. 3% salicylic acid and 6% benzoic acid (Whitfield's ointment).

Specific antifungal compounds include:

- Azole drugs such as imidazoles and triazoles, e.g. miconazole, econazole, ketoconazole, itraconazole and fluconazole.

- Allylamines, e.g. terbinafine.Terbinafine is a synthetic antifungal agent that is highly active against dermatophytes such as *Trichophyton*, *Microsporum* and *Epidermophyton floccosum* species. It is also active against moulds, dimorphic fungi and many yeasts of the genera *Pityrosporum*, *Candida* and *Rhodoturula*. The antimycotic activity of terbinafine is due to its interference with ergosterol biosynthesis, specifically its inhibition of fungal squalene epioxidase – squalene accumulates within the cell leading to concentrations that are toxic for the fungal cell.

- A miscellaneous group, including griseofulvin (oral), tolnaftate, amorolfine and cyclopiroxolamine.

Most antifungal drugs are fungistatic at therapeutic concentrations; terbinafine (topical and oral) is fungicidal – because of this and the fact that it enters skin and nail tissues very rapidly and is maintained there, it can be used for very short periods.

Topical therapy

This may be adequate for dermatophytosis other than nail infection – terbinafine cream, tolnaftate, imidazole, amorolfine or cyclopiroxolamine. Terbinafine cream takes about 1 week to kill the fungus, but the skin will take about 2–4 weeks to return to normal. The only topical agents giving some success in nail infection are amorolfine, cyclopiroxolamine and tioconazole.

Oral therapy

Griseofulvin, a fungistatic agent has been used for over 30 years at a dose of 10 mg/kg daily. For skin infection, 4–6 weeks' duration is needed and for nails the therapy is continued, until the nail returns to normal (success rates low).

Terbinafine is fungicidal at routine therapeutic concentrations and reaches adequate tissue levels in the most distal nail bed and nail plate within 3-4 weeks of the first dose. The early studies showed mycological cure rates of greater than 90% following only twelve weeks' treatment - dose 250 mg daily; subsequently similar cure rates have been produced with 6 weeks' therapy - compared with fungistatic oral griseofulvin which gives less than 50% success rates even if continuous treatment is given for over 1 year. Though preliminary usage of oral terbinafine in children has revealed no significant toxicity over a 56-day period, it is not currently recommended for use in children with onychomycosis. It is, however, interesting to note that pharmacokinetic studies have shown higher drug clearance in children compared with adults.

Oral itraconazole also gives high distal nail concentrations in studies using 200 mg daily. It has recently been recommended in a pulsed dose regime - 200 mg daily for 1 week in 4, with up to 6 pulses.

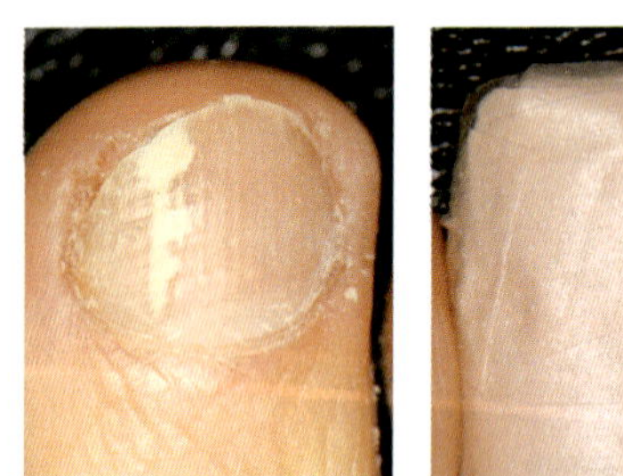
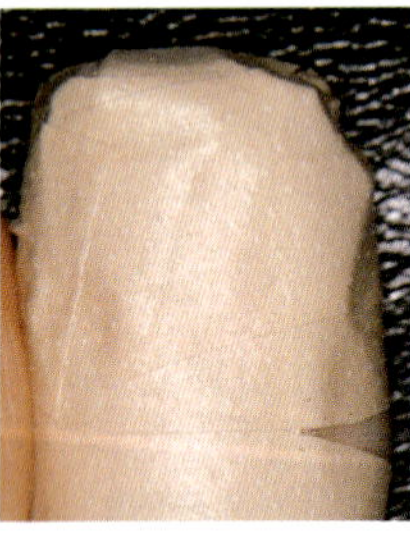
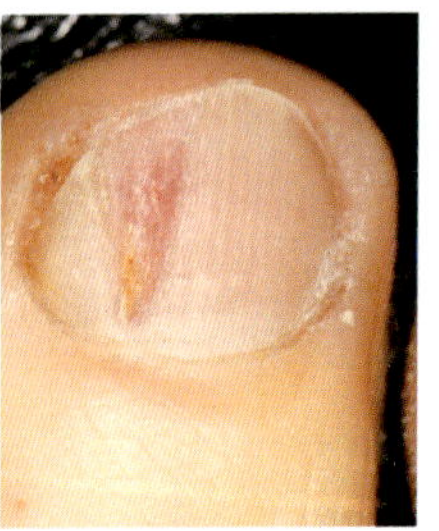

Figure 62
Urea paste nail avulsion: the affected nail is easily removed after 1 week of paste application. (Courtesy of Dr. R. Baran, Cannes, France.)

Urea avulsion may be useful to remove symptomatic affected nail – 40% urea paste is applied under occlusion for 1 week before cutting away the affected nail (Figure 62).

Viral warts

Plantar warts will often only require specific therapy if painful. Therapeutic principles include:

- Laissez-faire! Most remit within 3–6 months.
- Daily soaking in 3% formalin solution.
- Keratolytics – most preparations are based on salicylic acid as a paste – on plaster or in collodion. Up to 40% strength in some products; often combined with abrasion or paring.
- Cryosurgery – liquid nitrogen sprays most commonly used, i.e. from 5–30 seconds spray time, depending on site and size of lesion. Emla cream 2 hours before treatment may lessen discomfort.
- Bleomycin – solution applied to multiple surface puncture wounds.
- Cantharidin to induce cytolysis.
- Curettage and electrodesiccation under local anaesthetic.
- Carbon dioxide and pulsed die laser ablation.
- Local immunotherapy.
- Radiotherapy – rarely needed.
- Biopsy – if wart atypical, to exclude squamous carcinoma.

Ingrowing toenail

If conservative investigation, observation and antiseptic principles have failed, then a simple surgical operation is usually curative. Before proceeding to surgery:

- Check footwear – may be cause.
- Check foot and toe shape, and function.
- Check for onychomycosis.
- Check that nail trimming is being carried out correctly.
- Check the antiseptic or antibiotic treatment if chronic inflammation or infection is present.

The surgical procedure involved (Figure 63) is as follows:

- Ring-block local anaesthesia.
- Apply tourniquet.
- Avulse lateral ingrowing nail, approximately 25% of nail width.
- Apply yellow soft paraffin to nail folds.
- Apply 85% aqueous phenol to exposed matrix on an orange stick for 3 min.
- Double with 70% alcohol to neutralize the phenolic chemical cautery.
- The wound will remain moist for 2–3 weeks.
- Dress regularly until healing is completed.

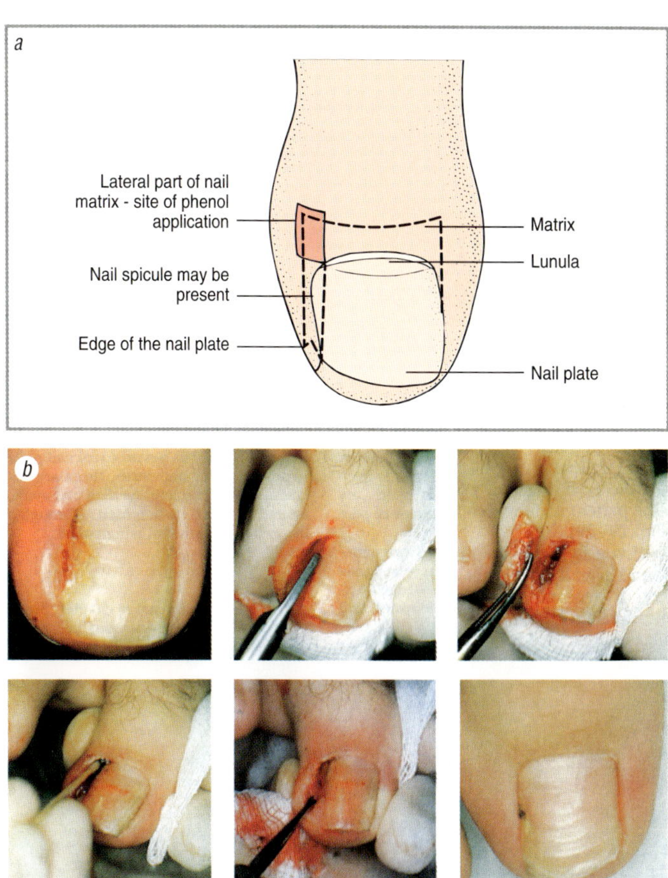

Figure 63
Ingrowing toenail: (a) showing matrix site to be phenolized, and (b) the operation details and result after healing. (Courtesy of Dr S Salasche, Tucson, USA.)

Index

A

B

C

D

E

F

G

H

I

J

K

L

M

N

O

P

R

S

T

U

V

W